# Naturally Occurring Small Molecules for Disease and Cancer Treatment

## Therapeutic Benefits in Combination Therapy

**Other Related Titles from World Scientific**

---

*Biodiversity, Natural Products and Cancer Treatment*
edited by Victor Kuete and Thomas Efferth
ISBN: 978-981-4583-50-3

*Cardioprotective Natural Products: Promises and Hopes*
edited by Goutam Brahmachari
ISBN: 978-981-3231-15-3

*Bioactive Natural Products: Opportunities and Challenges in Medicinal Chemistry*
edited by Goutam Brahmachari
ISBN: 978-981-4335-37-9

*Natural Products: Essential Resources for Human Survival*
edited by Yi-Zhun Zhu, Benny K-H Tan, Boon-Huat Bay and Chang-Hong Liu
ISBN: 978-981-270-498-6
ISBN: 978-981-3203-39-6 (pbk)

*Organic Synthesis via Examination of Selected Natural Products*
by David J Hart
ISBN: 978-981-4313-70-4

*Anticancer Properties of Fruits and Vegetables: A Scientific Review*
by Ajaikumar B Kunnumakkara
ISBN: 978-981-4508-88-9

# Naturally Occurring Small Molecules for Disease and Cancer Treatment

## Therapeutic Benefits in Combination Therapy

Wing Shing Ho

The Chinese University of Hong Kong, China

**World Scientific**

NEW JERSEY · LONDON · SINGAPORE · BEIJING · SHANGHAI · HONG KONG · TAIPEI · CHENNAI · TOKYO

*Published by*

World Scientific Publishing Co. Pte. Ltd.

5 Toh Tuck Link, Singapore 596224

*USA office:* 27 Warren Street, Suite 401-402, Hackensack, NJ 07601

*UK office:* 57 Shelton Street, Covent Garden, London WC2H 9HE

**Library of Congress Cataloging-in-Publication Data**

Names: Ho, Wing Shing, author.

Title: Naturally occurring small molecules for disease and cancer treatment :
    therapeutic benefits in combination therapy / by Wing Shing Ho.

Description: New Jersey : World Scientific, 2019. | Includes bibliographical references and index.

Identifiers: LCCN 2018052413 | ISBN 9789814525626 (hardcover : alk. paper)

Subjects: | MESH: Neoplasms--drug therapy | Drugs, Chinese Herbal--therapeutic use |
    Antineoplastic Agents--therapeutic use | Small Molecule Libraries | Drug Therapy, Combination

Classification: LCC RC271.C5 | NLM QZ 267 | DDC 616.99/4061--dc23

LC record available at https://lccn.loc.gov/2018052413


**British Library Cataloguing-in-Publication Data**

A catalogue record for this book is available from the British Library.

For any available supplementary material, please visit
https://www.worldscientific.com/worldscibooks/10.1142/8916#t=suppl

# TABLE OF CONTENTS

*About the Author* ...................................................................................*vii*

*Preface*...................................................................................................*ix*

*Acknowledgments*...................................................................................*xi*

**1.** Principles of Pharmacology of Cancer Drug Treatment........................1

**2.** Plant Molecules ...............................................................................16

**3.** Herbal Medicines .............................................................................30

**4.** Therapeutic Uses of Small Molecules ......................................................41

**5.** Mechanism of Action .........................................................................47

**6.** Integration and Control of the Human Body During Treatment.......61

**7.** Cytotoxic Plant Molecules and Immunopharmacology ......................75

**8.** Potential Beneficial Effects of Plant Products.........................................86

**9.** Adverse Drug Reactions........................................................................96

**10.** Treatment of Cancer with Natural Products ......................................107

**11.** Pharmaceutical Development of Potential Cancer Drugs................123

*Appendix*

*(chemical structures of phytochemical compounds. The reactive moiety/atom is highlighted in color.)*

**I.** Chapter 2 .................................................................................... 131

**II.** Chapter 5 .................................................................................. 136

**III.** Chapter 7 ................................................................................. 137

**IV.** Chapter 9 ................................................................................. 139

*Index* ................................................................................................ *143*

**Professor Wing Shing Ho** obtained his BSc. from The University of Alberta and MA, PhD in the field of biological chemistry from the State University of New York at Buffalo in 1981 and 1985, respectively. He completed his postdoctoral work at the Center for Human Toxicology, University of Utah until 1992, and has since returned to Hong Kong to take on the position of associate professor at the School of Life Sciences, The Chinese University of Hong Kong. His research interests are in the area of bio-active plant chemical compounds beneficial to humans and medical nutrition therapy and detoxification. He has been granted three patents on herbal medicine and has also applied for a number of patents. Prof. Ho has published over 100 papers in several international journals.

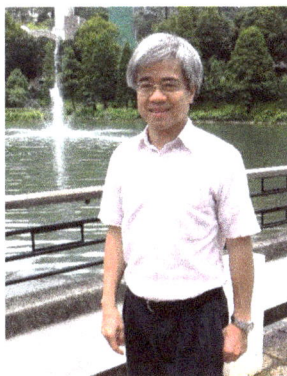

# PREFACE

Herbal medicine uses plants or mixtures of plant extracts and aims to restore your body's ability to protect, regulate, and heal itself. It is based on the whole-body approach to help regulate the body functions including mental and emotional states. Recent development on herbal medicine promises to offer new hope for cancer therapy. Novel phytochemicals with multi-arrays of pharmacological activities including anticancer medicinal properties have been reported. New drugs are developed based on the active compounds of plants. This book covers recent studies on the health benefits and pharmacological actions of active compounds of herbal medicines in combination of drugs in cancer therapy. The development of active compounds from herbal medicine in combination with drugs in the context of cancers and the diseases shows great promise. The biological actions of the naturally occurring active phytochemicals at the molecular and cellular levels and their benefits with drugs are discussed. The book provides insightful information on how phytochemicals can be integrated with other drugs for cancer treatment. It is planned to use conventional icons to explain the main biological actions of phytochemicals in practical applications as checkpoint regulators or inhibitors of signaling pathways, which are associated with a variety of biological process. The important aspects of the integrated medicines including health benefits and the drawback of phytochemicals are discussed. The book also includes illustrations to show the relevant interactions in our body. Other important issues related to phytochemical actions of herbal medicine are also described. Prescribing drugs is used to compare the phytochemical actions in *in vivo* study.

This book has been designed for scientists who are interested in herbal medicine and its development. It would be useful to related healthcare professions. The book context would enable readers to get a better understanding and appreciation of herbal medicines in combination with or without drugs in personalized medicine for treatment of various diseases.

# ACKNOWLEDGMENTS

The author would like to express his heart-felt gratitude to his postgraduate students and staff members who have helped him at the time of writing and the technical assistance in preparation of the materials. Special thanks to my wife, Hiu Yin, and two sons, Kam Yuen and Kam Hang, for their patience and understanding of the work load that took up a lot of time.

# PRINCIPLES OF PHARMACOLOGY OF CANCER DRUG TREATMENT

## Introduction

Herbal medicines have been used for treatment of diseases in China for thousands of years. The composition of phytochemicals in herbal medicines varies among different plant species. Phytochemicals are useful to characterize their medicinal properties of herbs. Phytochemicals may have multi-arrays of other biological significance, e.g., polyphenols, flavonoids, saponins, or carotenoids. Some of these phytochemicals are established as essential nutrients in foods and has been reported in various plants. There are at least 150 kinds of naturally occurring saponins that have been found to possess anti-cancer properties and more than 11 distinguished classes of saponins including dammaranes, tirucallanes, lupanes, hopanes, oleananes, taraxasteranes, ursanes, cycloartanes, lanostanes, cucurbitanes, and steroids.[1] Due to differences in their chemical structures, saponins can display anti-tumorigenic effects on cancer cells yet active phytochemicals from herbal medicine are not easily identified. Although a number of active phytochemicals have been reported, their chemistry and reactivity and the pharmacological activities and mechanism of action and structure–function relationships at the molecular and cellular levels remain to be explored. Some special saponins with strong antitumor effects have been exhibited. Ginsenosides which are dammaranes are shown to exhibit anti-angiogenesis and inhibiting metastasis. In addition, Dioscin, one of the steroidal saponins, and its aglycone diosgenin are inducers of cell cycle arrest and apoptosis. Table 1.1 shows the medicinal properties of saponins.

**Table 1.1** Medical application of selected saponins

| Family | Species | Saponins | Cancer | Ref. |
|---|---|---|---|---|
| **Agavaceae** | *Agave utahensis* | Chlorogenin hexasaccharide | HL-60 | Yokosuka et al.[2], Xu et al.[3] |
| **Alliaceae** | *Allium macrostemon* Bunge | Macrostemo-noside O, P, Q, and R | HepG2, MCF-7 | Yang et al.[4] |
| **Aslepiadceae** | *Cynanchum auriculatum* | Wilfoside C3N | A549 | Liu et al.[5], Kim et al.[6] |
| **Asparagaceae** | *Asparagus gobicus* | Asparanin A | HepG2 | Yang et al.[7], Wang et al.[8] |
| **Dioscoreaceae** | Disscorea | (25S)-spirost-5-en-3$\beta$ | L929, HeLa | Liu et al.[9], Gonzalez et al.[10] |
| **Dracaenaceae** | Nam ginseng | Namonins | HT-1080, BL6 | [11], Tran et al.[12] |
| **Liliaceae** | *Polygonatum sibiricum Camassia cusickii* | Neosibirico-sides A-D TGHS-1 and 2 | MCF-7 P388 | Sy et al.[13], Ahn et al.[14] |
| **Solanaceae** | *Solanum torvum Solanum indicum* L. | Torvosides M Dioscin | HepG2, MCF-7, Colo-205, HSC-2, human fibroblasts | Nartowska et al.[15], Lu et al.[16] |

Infectious diseases which are infected by microorganisms such as protozoa are of major health concern worldwide. The incidence of the disease has increased since the emergence of AIDS and Ebola diseases. In the absence of a vaccine and satisfactory drugs, there is an urgent need for novel drugs to replace or to supplement those in current use. Herbal medicines are undoubtedly a valuable source of new medicinal agents. However, active phytochemicals remain to be identified and characterized. Herbal extracts and chemically defined molecules of natural origin show various medicinal activities. It also includes about three hundred compounds isolated from higher plants and microorganisms, which are classified into chemical groups with specific biologic activity.[17]

Many herbal medicine-derived compounds display significant effects on body functions. They can be good candidates for drug development for treatment of various diseases including rheumatism, asthma, and atherosclerosis. Many herbal extracts and the respective active compounds isolated from natural resources for the treatment of various diseases have been reported yet individual active compounds may not display the same activity *in vivo*. Herbal extracts are reported to exhibit anti-viral activity against herpes simplex virus (HSV), both the types 1 and 2.[18] Therefore, medicinal plants can be a good source for drug development. However, the bioactive anti-HSV molecules from the plant extracts need to be identified and tested. The mechanism of actions of the potential active anti-HSV molecule(s) requires tedious research work. Similar methodology for isolation, purification, and characterization of potential phytochemicals from other herbal medicines can be used. The most potent molecule(s) and their analogues need to undergo preclinical and toxicity evaluations before synthesis of a large amount of the bioactive molecules for medical applications. In another approach such as genomics, gene expression profiling could help to identify molecular targets of the biological activity of the active natural products that would facilitate the gene-based drug development.

## Sesquiterpene

Apart from this, another common class of phytochemicals, Sesquiterpene lactones have been reported as the major phytoconstituents of *Saussurea costus*. Different pharmacological experiments in a number of *in vitro* and *in vivo* models have demonstrated the medicinal properties of *S. costus* with anti-inflammatory, anti-ulcer, anti-cancer, and hepato-protective activities.[19]

## Flavonoids

Flavonoids are a large family of polyphenols present in herbal medicines. Six major subclasses of flavonoids, namely anthocyanidins, flavan-3-ols, flavonols, flavanones, flavones, and isoflavones.[20,21] Table 1.2 shows the source

**Table 1.2** Common plant flavonoids[20,21]

| Flavonoid Subclass | Dietary Flavonoids (aglycones) | Some Common Food Sources |
|---|---|---|
| Anthocyanidins | Cyanidin, Delphinidin, Malvidin, Pelargonidin, Peonidin, Petunidin | Red, blue, and purple berries; red and purple grapes; red wine |
| Flavan-3-ols | Monomers (Catechins): (+)-Catechin, (−)-Epicatechin, (−)-Epigallocatechin, (+)-Gallocatechin; and their gallate derivatives | Teas (white, green, and oolong), grapes, berries, apples |
| | Dimers and Polymers: Proanthocyanidins# | Apples, berries, cocoa-based products, red grapes, red wine |
| | Theaflavins, Thearubigins | Black tea |
| Flavonols | Isorhamnetin, Kaempferol, Myricetin, Quercetin | Onions, scallions, kale, broccoli, apples, berries, teas |
| Flavones | Apigenin, Luteolin, Baicalein, Chrysin | Parsley, thyme, celery, hot peppers |
| Flavanones | Eriodictyol, Hesperetin, Naringenin | Citrus fruit and juices, e.g., oranges, grapefruits, lemons |
| Isoflavones | Daidzein, Genistein, Glycitein, Biochanin A, Formononetin | Soybeans, soy foods, legumes |

of some common plant flavonols. Flavonols are the most commonly found in plants and vegetables and fruit. The biochemical properties of flavonoids influence their disposition. Their metabolites exert biological activities relevant to the health benefits in human health. Many of the biological effects of flavonoids are related to their ability to modulate cell-signaling processes and cell growth. In addition, flavonoids are shown to exhibit multi-arrays of pharmacologic activities including anti-inflammatory, anti-thrombogenic, anti-diabetic, and anti-cancer. Previous studies suggest that consumption of flavan-3-ols and anthocyanidins can exert therapeutic effects on cardio-vascular disorders and type 2 diabetes mellitus. However, only a limited number of studies has reported the anti-cancer activities of flavonoids in humans but higher intake of soy isoflavones appeared to be associated with reduction in cancer risks of breast in women and prostate cancer in men. Yet the health benefits of flavonoids remain to be further investigated.

## Phytochemicals from cruciferous vegetables

Cruciferous vegetables, such as broccoli and cabbage, contain various sulfur-containing compounds called glucosinolates. Isothiocyanates are biologically active products of glucosinolates.[22] For example, broccoli is a good source of glucoraphanin, the glucosinolate precursor of sulforaphane (SFN), and sinigrin, the glucosinolate precursor of allyl isothiocyanate (AITC).[23-26] Glucosinolates are present in medicinal plants. Watercress is a rich source of gluconasturtiin, the precursor of phenethyl isothiocyanate (PEITC), while garden cress is rich in glucotropaeolin, the precursor of ben-zyl isothiocyanate (BITC). At present, scientists are interested in synthesis of the glucosinolate analogues that exhibit cancer-preventive activities. When cruciferous vegetables are chopped or chewed, myrosinase can interact with glucosinolates and release isothiocyanates from their precursors (Figure 1.1).

The myrosinase activity of human intestinal bacteria allows for some formation and absorption of isothiocyanates.[27-29] Like most other herbal medicines, cruciferous vegetables are good sources of a variety of phyto-chemicals that may work synergistically to help prevent cancer.[22,28,30,31] Cruciferous vegetable or herbal medicines intake and cancer risk in humans can be related. Diets that are generally rich in beneficial phytochemicals

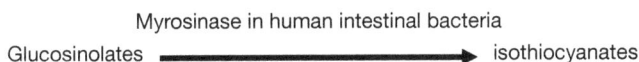

Myrosinase in human intestinal bacteria

Glucosinolates ⟶ isothiocyanates

**Figure 1.1** Transformation of glucosinolates in human gastrointestinal tract.

like those characteristic with high glucosinolate content can be cancer preventive.[31] Glucosinolate hydrolysis products could help prevent cancer by enhancing the elimination of carcinogens before they can damage DNA, or by altering cell-signaling pathways in ways that help prevent normal cells from being transformed into cancerous cells.[30,31] Some glucosinolate hydrolysed products may alter the metabolism or activity of hormones like estrogen in ways that inhibit the development of hormone-sensitive cancers. However, a very high intake of cruciferous vegetables, such as cabbage have been found to cause thyroid disorders in animals.[32,33] The hydrolysis of some glucosinolates found in cruciferous vegetables (e.g., progoitrin) may yield a compound known as goitrin, which has been found to interfere with thyroid hormone biosynthesis. The hydrolysis of another class of glucosinolates, known as indole glucosinolates, results in the release of thiocyanate ions, which can compete with iodine for uptake by the thyroid gland. Increased exposure to thiocyanate ions from cruciferous vegetable consumption or from cigarette smoking does not appear to increase the risk of hypothyroidism unless accompanied by iodine deficiency.

There is an increasing interest in exploitation and use of herbal medicines for treatment of various ailments worldwide. Traditional Chinese Medicine (TCM) especially in specific herbal formulations are effective in treatment of chronic diseases. It is believed that individual phytochemicals in the formulations interact to produce the health benefits.

Naturally occurring plant chemicals can influence the biochemical activities in different ways. The health benefits of anti-cancer phytochemicals may include the following activities:

   (i)   Induction of apoptosis
  (ii)   Anti-cancer
 (iii)   Anti-inflammation
  (iv)   Regulation of the immune system
   (v)   Modulation of oxidative damage to cells.

Although many phytochemicals have been identified and more are being isolated and characterized in plants and organisms, the potential of phytochemicals in herbal medicines remains to be investigated.

Table 1.3 lists some of the phytochemicals that are present in vegetables and fruits. This kind of phytochemicals is also found in herbal medicines but at different concentrations. The concentration difference and

**Table 1.3** Some of the phytochemicals are commonly found in vegetables and fruits

| Phytochemical(s) | Source | Health Benefits |
|---|---|---|
| Carotenoids (such as beta-carotene, lycopene, lutein, and zeaxanthin) | Red, orange, and green fruits and vegetables, e.g., broccoli, carrots, lettuce, sweet potatoes, apricots, cantaloupe, oranges, and watermelon | Anti-oxidants |
| Flavonoids (such as anthocyanins and quercetin) | Apples, citrus fruits, and vegetables, e.g., onions, soybeans, and soy products, e.g., tofu, soy milk, coffee, and tea | Anti-inflammatory and anti-cancer; enhancement of liver functions |
| Indoles and glucosinolates (sulforaphane); Isothiocyanates | Cruciferous vegetables, e.g., broccoli, cabbage, cauliflower, and Brussels sprouts | Reduction of oxidative stress due to carcinogens |
| Inositol (phytic acid) | Vegetables: corn, oats, rice, rye and wheat, nuts, soybeans, and soy products (tofu, soy milk, edamame, etc.) | Inhibition of cancer cell growth |
| Isoflavones (daidzein and genistein) | Soybeans and soy products (tofu, soy milk, edamame, etc.) | Inhibition of cancer growth |
| Polyphenols (such as ellagic acid and resveratrol) | Green tea, grapes, wine, berries, citrus fruits, apples, whole grains, and peanuts | Anti-inflammation and anti-oxidative |
| Terpenes (such as perillyl alcohol, limonene, and carnosol) | Cherries, citrus fruit peel, and rosemary | Anti-viral and anti-oxidative |

composition of individual phytochemicals between plant species make a difference in their health benefits.

Nowadays, there has been a propensity to application of natural phytochemicals in diverse intrinsic rich sources of agricultural produce such as fruits, leaves, branches as well as roots of different plants because of existence of substituents with bioactive potentials. Many medicinal herbs compositions contribute to remedial specifications. Plants are classified by geographical territory that makes a significant difference in herbal properties. The various herbaceous infusions, such as antidiabetic, anti-carcinogenic, antimicrobial, and antioxidant show diverse functions.[34]

# Chinese herbal medicine

Chinese herbal medicine is part of a whole system of medicine called Traditional Chinese Medicine (TCM). TCM aims to restore the balance of your Qi (pronounced chee). TCM practitioners believe that Qi is the flow of energy in your body, and is essential for good health. Chinese herbalists use medicinal plants according to their medicinal properties that can affect a particular part of the body or energy channel.

TCM includes:

- Herbal prescription
- Acupuncture
- Massage therapy
- Traditional breathing and movement exercises include qi gong (pronounced chee goong) and tai chi (pronounced tie chee).

# Herbal medicine for the treatment of atherosclerosis

Research into atherosclerosis has led to discovery of herbal medicine yet TCM has been widely used in China as well as other Asian countries for the treatment of cardiovascular diseases for hundreds of years; however, the mechanisms of action of TCM in the treatment of atherosclerosis remains sketchy. The mechanism of atherogenesis and antiatherogenic herbal compounds were reported yet the detail of its activity is lacking. However, the study provides a platform to build a bridge between TCM and cellular and molecular cardiovascular medicine.[35]

Herbal medicines commonly used for cardiovascular diseases include Danshen which has been commonly used in TCM for treatment of a variety of diseases, including coronary artery disease, acute ischemic stroke, hyperlipidemia, chronic renal failure, chronic hepatitis, and Alzheimer's disease without adverse effects. Recent studies have shown that cryptotanshinone not only possesses the potential for treatment and prevention of the cardiovascular diseases but it also displayed anticancer activity.[35,36]

# Medicinal plants are an essential part of TCM

The ancient complex therapy theory is considered today as one of the most complete complementary medicine system. TCM listings included in Chinese Materia Medica cover more than 1500 plants and a great number of composite preparations.[37] Several TCM herbs have been included into European Pharmacopoeia and the listings are being increased. The efficiency of TCM is based on an organism's natural healing power and the ability to restore the energy homoeostasis. It is agreed that the mechanism of the functional activities is interacting with redox balance and reduction of oxidative stress. Over hundreds of crude herbs, extracts, and isolated compounds have been screened for their antioxidant properties *in vitro* and *in vivo*.[37] The anti-oxidant activity of TCM contributes to their therapeutic and preventive benefits. With TCM and food plants, various classes of antioxidant compounds such as polyphenols or terpenoids have been identified. These anti-oxidants can remove reactive oxygen species.

# TCM as complementary medicine for treatment of disease

In Chinese medicine, any health problem is a consequence of the disorientation and imbalance of "Yin-Yang" of which the body naturally can sustain harmony and integrity under healthy conditions. Traditional Chinese Medical Theory dictates that all of the energies in the body must be balanced relative to one another all the time in order to maintain good health and homeostasis. The Yin (substance) must be balanced with the Yang (energy), the organs must harmoniously work and coordinate together to protect the body from any changes, and the Shen (emotions) must stay low and calm.[38–41]

Yin is substance to be maintained at high spirit. However, it is necessary to first maintain the Yin so that the Yang energy can be efficiently used all the time. There is no absolute Yin, or absolute Yang. Yet there is a bit of Yin in Yang, and there is a bit of Yang in Yin. Also, Yin and Yang should be flowing effectively in the body which cannot be suspended at any one time, otherwise the body experiences some kind of health problems. This is demonstrated in the body by twisted joints; first, the injured joint is getting hot and inflamed. As this Yang condition transforms to Yin, the inflammation becomes obvious and swelling appears around the injured joint and goes down and the injured joint becomes stiff. All these disease patterns will pass through Yin and Yang phases until treated with appropriate medicines.

The use of TCM is based on the concept of Yin and Yang. Yin and Yang represent the fundamental duality in the universe or in our system in which a duality is ultimately adjusted to harmony. Yin and Yang are complementary. The body may have a Yin-Yang imbalance but everyone has both qualities.

Harmony of body functions needs to be maintained between these Yin and Yang qualities and any imbalance can be modulated with TCM. Yin is like blood, fluids, and tissue in the body. Yang is the action potential, Qi, and heat in the body. Qi (pronounced "chee") is generally thought of as the vital driving force within our bodies. Qi in its Yang form is responsible for thermodynamics and balance of the human functions. Chinese medicines are to balance Yin and Yang when they are deficient or imbalance. No one person is completely with Yin or Yang; rather, one would be diagnosed for any imbalances and patterns. One organ system may have Yang excess while another organ system in the same body can have Yang Deficiency.

Many people recognize that they often feel cold or Yang Deficient and an attempt is to take a Yang tonic by itself only to develop Deficient Heat signs such as afternoon or evening sweats or fevers. In Chinese medicine, it is always important to build Yin before attempting to build Yang because your body lacks the substance to support the Yin which is just like fire. The kidney plays an important role in energizing the system. This is why kidney tonics are employed when reinforcing Yin and Yang qualities in the body.

Each individual can encounter different degrees of deficiency and imbalances in any one organ or tissues at any time. Because of this, the use of Yin and Yang tonics varies from person to person. When body, mind, and spirit are harmonized, one can only then stay in a balance of Yin-Yang and a good health status without health problems.

# Development of tumors and cancers

It is believed that cancers are a result of accumulations of "Qi", moisture and blood that cannot be circulating effectively in the body.[39,40] The morbid tissues subsequently cause disturbance in normal circulation of blood and lymph. Therefore, treatment of these disturbances with TCM would aim at modulating these crucial factors, namely, "Qi", moisture and blood and eliminate the health problems.

It is believed that the relationship between blood and its circulation is important in ameliorating the deficiency in Yin-Yang and its balance in the body. When there is insufficient "Ying Qi", the distribution of "Qi" is significantly interrupted. Consequently, therapeutic measures are needed to remove the obstruction and restore efficient blood circulation. Chinese medicines such as angelica, salvia, and millettia are to treat both deficiency and stasis because they can enhance blood circulation.

Deficiency in "Qi" and blood would cause problems in removing the toxic metabolites in the body. For example, lung cancer may result from abnormal patterns such as liver "Qi" that causes imbalance of Yin-Yang in the lung due to "Yang" deficiency, phlegm stagnation and blood stagnation and "Yin" deficiency due to lung heat, "Qi" and blood deficiency. Depending on the patterns of deficiency, therapies with Chinese medicines are administered according to the pathological patterns and the health status of the patient. Herbal formulas relieve stagnation by using "Qi" and blood-activating herbs and antidote toxins. Anti-cancer herbs are used to dissolve these pathogenic entities.

# Acupuncture for treatment of cancer

Acupuncture can be used to enhance blood circulation as well. The common cancer therapy such as radiation and chemotherapy would cause accumulation of toxins due to drug toxicity. Surgery would interrupt blood circulation in some tissues. Appropriate Chinese medicines are especially effective to invigorate the "Qi" and to enhance blood circulation. Consequently, the use of TCM could help modulate stress, enhance host defense mechanism and to boost the immune system to reduce infection, and suppress the progression of tumors. The combination of TCM and acupuncture is the common complementary method for management of cancer for thousands of years in China and other Asian countries. Chinese medicines can be used alone or in combination with Western drugs for cancer therapy.[42–45] The use of TCM and drug combination has become the common practice in China.[42,43] The use of herbs in combinations with anticancer drugs was reported to modulate the chemoresistance as a result of repeated use of the anticancer drug. Ginseng is widely used in countries worldwide as an adjuvant for cancer therapy. It is used as a dietary or an herbal supplement in European and Asian countries. Although Ginseng consumption is not limited for in cancer patients, its benefit in treatment of diseases is well recognized. In addition, Ginseng exerts a chemopreventive action against cancer.[46]

Herbal medicines become the alternative choice in complementary medicine. While Western medicine can inhibit the cancer growth, TCM supports and restores the functions of vital organs due to drug toxicity. The quality of life of patients can therefore be improved.

## Recent development on TCM

Over the last decades, integrated medicine has become a common practice in treatment of various diseases. The combination of drugs and Chinese medicines are to enhance the therapeutic effects without compromising the efficacy of drugs and at the time Chinese medicines help modulate the side effects of drugs. Cancer patients usually show symptoms of deficiency in "Qi", blood and functions of vital organs including liver and kidney. Accumulation of toxins may worsen the health conditions and the immune functions. Tonic treatment would be the top choice strategy in treatment of cancer patients.

Chinese herbal medicines have become increasingly popular among cancer patients. Chinese herbal medicines are used as adjuvant therapy under the guidance of experienced Chinese medicine practitioners. However, interactions between herbal medicines and cancer drugs can occur due to health status of cancer patients; thus, the herb–drug interactions can cause otherwise harmful effects on patients.

Nowadays, it has become increasingly important for cancer patients to adopt some complementary protocols in order to reduce cytotoxicity of cancer drugs. In women with advanced breast cancer, co-administration of garlic supplement reduced the clearance of docetaxol.[47,48] The study alleviated cytotoxicity due to cancer drugs-induced liver toxicity. Most cancer drugs are substrates of P-glycoprotein, and can cause multidrug resistance associated proteins and other transporters. Induction and inhibition of the drug-metabolizing enzymes and transporters may affect efficacy of therapeutic drugs. Therefore, the selection of appropriate herbal medicines and the cancer drug for cancer therapy is important to avoid health hazard.

# References

1.  Man, S., Gao, W., Zhang, Y., Huang, L., and Liu, C. (2010). Chemical study and medical application of saponins as anti-cancer agents. *Fitoterapia*. 81: 703–714.
2.  Yokosuka, A., Jitsuno, M., Yui, S., Yamazaki, M., and Mimaki, Y. (2009). Steroidal glycosides from *Agave utahensis* and their cytotoxic activity. *J Nat Prod*. 72: 1399–1404.
3.  Xu, Y., Chiu, J.F., He, Q.Y., and Chen, F. (2009). Tubeimoside-1 exerts cytotoxicity in HeLa cells through mitochondrial dysfunction and endoplasmic reticulum stress pathways. *J Proteome Res*. 8: 1585–1593.
4.  Yang, M.F., Li, Y.Y., Gao, X.P., Li, B.G., and Zhang, G.L. (2004). Steroidal saponins from *Myriopteron extensum* and their cytotoxic activity. *Planta Med*. 70: 556–560.
5.  Liu, W., Huang, X.F., Qi, Q., *et al.* (2009). Asparanin A induces G(2)/M cell cycle arrest and apoptosis in human hepatocellular carcinoma HepG2 cells. *Biochem Biophys Res Commun*. 381: 700–705.
6.  Kim, G.S., Kim, H.T., and Seong, J.D. (2005). Cytotoxic steroidal saponins from the rhizomes of *Asparagus oligoclonos*. *J Nat Prod*. 68: 766–768.
7.  Yang, C.X., Huang, S.S., Yang, X.P., and Jia, Z.J. (2004). Nor-lignans and steroidal saponins from *Asparagus gobicus*. *Planta Med*. 70: 446–451.
8.  Wang, S.L., Cai, B., and Cui, C.B. (2003). Apoptosis of human chronic myeloid leukemia k562 cell induced by prosapogenin B of dioscin (P.B) in vitro. *Chin J Cancer*. 22: 795–800.
9.  Liu, H.W., Hu, K., and Zhao, Q.C. (2002). Bioactive saponins from *Dioscorea futschauensis*. *Pharmazie*. 57: 570–572.
10. Gonzalez, A.G., Hernandez, J.C., and Leon, F. (2003). Steroidal saponins from the bark of *Dracaena draco* and their cytotoxic activities. *J Nat Prod*. 66: 793–798.
11. Dong, M.X., Meng, .Z.F., Kuerban, K., Qi, F.L., Liu, J.Y, Wei, Y.X., Wang, Q., Jiang, S.S., Feng, M.Q., and Ye, L. (2018). Diosgenin promotes antitumor immunity and PD-1 antibody efficacy against melanoma by regulating intestinal microbiota. *Cell Death & Death*. Volume: 9. Article Number: 1039. DOI: 10.1038/s41419-018-1099-3.
12. Tran, Q.L., Tezuka, Y., and Banskota, A.H. (2001). New spirostanol steroids and steroidal saponins from roots and rhizomes of *Dracaena angustifolia* and their antiproliferative activity. *J Nat Prod*. 64: 1127–1132.
13. Sy, L.K., Yan, S.C., Lok, C.N., Man, R.Y., and Che, C.M. (2008). Timosaponin A-III induces autophagy preceding mitochondria-mediated apoptosis in HeLa cancer cells. *Cancer Res*. 68: 10229–10237.
14. Ahn, M.J., Kim, C.Y., and Yoon, K.D. (2006). Steroidal saponins from the rhizomes of *Polygonatum sibiricum*. *J Nat Prod*. 69: 360–364.
15. Nartowska, J., Sommer, E., Pastewka, K., Sommer, S., and Skopinska-Rozewska, E. (2004). Anti-angiogenic activity of convallamaroside, the steroidal saponin isolated from the rhizomes and roots of *Convallaria majalis* L. *Acta Pol Pharm*. 61: 279–282.
16. Lu, Y., Luo, J., Huang, X., and Kong, L. (2009). Four new steroidal glycosides from *Solanum torvum* and their cytotoxic activities. *Steroids*. 74: 95–101.

17. Tareq, M., Khana, H., Ather, A., Thompson, K.D., and Gambari, R. (2005). Extracts and molecules from medicinal plants against herpes simplex viruses. *Antiviral Res.* 67: 107–119.

18. Rocha, L.G., Almeida, J.R., Macêdo, R.O., and Barbosa-Filhob, J.M. (2005). A review of natural products with antileishmanial activity. *Phytomedicine.* 12: 514–535.

19. Pandey, M.M., Rastogi, S., Kumar, A., and Rawat, S. (2007). *Saussurea costus*: botanical, chemical and pharmacological review of an ayurvedic medicinal plant. *J Ethnopharmacol.* 110: 379–390.

20. Manach, C., Scalbert, A., Morand, C., Remesy, C., and Jimenez, L. (2004). Polyphenols: food sources and bioavailability. *Am J Clin Nutr.* 79(5): 727–747.

21. Xiao, J., Kai, G., Yamamoto, K., and Chen, X. (2013). Advance in dietary polyphenols as α-glucosidases inhibitors: a review on structure-activity relationship aspect. *Crit Rev Food Sci Nutr.* 53(8): 818–836.

22. Zhang, Y. (2004). Cancer-preventive isothiocyanates: measurement of human exposure and mechanism of action. *Mutat Res.* 555(1–2): 173–190.

23. Hecht, S.S. (2004). Chemoprevention by isothiocyanates. In: Kelloff GJ, Hawk ET, and Sigman CC, eds. *Promising Cancer Chemopreventive Agents, Volume 1: Cancer Chemopreventive Agents.* Totowa, NJ: Humana Press: 21–35.

24. Zhao, Y.L., Hu, X.Q., Zuo, X.Y., and Wang, M.F. (2018). Chemopreventive effects of some popular phytochemicals on human colon cancer: a review. *Food & Function.* 9(9): 4548–4568. DOI: 10.1039/c8fo00850g.

25. Holst, B., and Williamson, G. (2004). A critical review of the bioavailability of glucosinolates and related compounds. *Nat Prod Rep.* 21(3): 425–447.

26. Meng, J., Cheung, W.M., Yu, V., Zhou, Y., Tong, P.H., and Ho, W.S. (2014). Antiproliferative activities of sinigrin on carcinogen-induced hepatotoxicity in rats. *PLOS ONE.* 9(10): e110145.

27. Aires, A., Mota, V.R., Saavedra, M.J., Rosa, E.A.S., and Bennett, R.N. (2009). The antimicrobial effects of glucosinolates and their respective enzymatic hydrolysis products on bacteria isolated from the human intestinal tract. *J Appl Microbiol.* 106: 2086–2095.

28. van Poppel, G., Verhoeven, D.T., Verhagen, H., and Goldbohm, R.A. (1999). Brassica vegetables and cancer prevention. Epidemiology and mechanisms. *Adv Exp Med Biol.* 472: 159–168.

29. Verhoeven, D.T., Goldbohm, R.A., van Poppel, G., Verhagen, H., and van den Brand, P.A. (1996). Epidemiological studies on brassica vegetables and cancer risk. *Cancer Epidemiol Biomarkers Prev.* 5(9): 733–748.

30. Liu, R.H. (2004). Potential synergy of phytochemicals in cancer prevention: mechanism of action. *J Nutr.* 134(Suppl 12): 3479S–3485S.

31. McNaughton, S.A., and Marks, G.C. (2003). Development of a food composition database for the estimation of dietary intakes of glucosinolates, the biologically active constituents of cruciferous vegetables. *Br J Nutr.* 90(3): 687–697.

32. Fenwick, G.R., Heaney, R.K., and Mullin, W.J. (1983). Glucosinolates and their breakdown products in food and food plants. *Crit Rev Food Sci Nutr.* 18(2): 123–201.

33. Chu, M., and Seltzer, T.F. (2010). Myxedema coma induced by ingestion of raw bok choy. *N Engl J Med.* 362(20): 1945–1946.

34. Farzaneh, V., and Carvalho, I.S. (2015). A review of the health benefit potentials of herbal plant infusions and their mechanism of actions. *Ind Crops Prod.* 65: 247–258.

35. Liu, Q., Li, J.P., Hartstone-Rose, A., *et al.* (2015). Chinese herbal compounds for the treatment of atherosclerosis: experimental evidence and mechanisms. *Evid Based Complement Altern Med.* 2015: 1–15.

36. Chen, W., Lu, Y., Chen, G., and Huang, S. (2013). Molecular evidence of cryptotanshinone for treatment and prevention of human cancer. *Anticancer Agents Med Chem.* 7: 979–987.

37. Matkowski, A., Jamiołkowska-Kozlowska, W., and Nawrot, I. (2013). Chinese medicinal herbs as source of antioxidant compounds—where tradition meets the future. *Curr Med Chem.* 20(8): 984–1004.

38. Benefield, H., and Korngold, E. (2003). Chinese medicine and cancer care. *Altern Ther.* 9(5): 38–52.

39. Guorui, T. (1981). *The Use of Tonics in China—Past, Present, and Future.* Beijing: Academy of Traditional Chinese Medicine.

40. Porkert, J. (1974). *The Theoretical Foundations of Chinese Medicine.* MIT Press.

41. Chen, J.K., and Chen, T.T. (2003). *Chinese Medical Herbology and Pharmacology.* Art of Medicine Press.

42. Kan, S., Cheung, W.M., Zhou, Y., and Ho, W.S. (2014). Enhancement of doxorubicin cytotoxicity by tanshinone IIA in HepG2 human hepatoma cells. *Planta Med.* 80: 70–77.

43. Chen, S., Wang, Z., Huang, Y., *et al.* (2014). Ginseng and anticancer drug combination to improve cancer chemotherapy: a critical review. *Evid Based Complement Altern Med.* 14: 1–13.

44. Che, C.T., Wang, Z., Chow, M.S.S., and Lam, C.W.K. (2013). Herb combination for therapeutic enhancement and advancement: theory, practice and future perspectives. *Molecules.* 18: 5125–5141.

45. Qi, F., Li, A., and Inagaki, Y. (2010). Chinese herbal medicines as adjuvant treatment during chemo- or radio-therapy for cancer. *BioSci Trends.* 4(6): 297–307.

46. Yun, T., and Choi, S. (1995). Preventive effect of ginseng intake against various human cancers: a case-control study on 1987 pairs. *Cancer Epidemiol Biomarkers Prev.* 4(4): 401–408.

47. Kim, S.M., Lee, S.Y., Cho, J.S., *et al.* (2010). Combination of ginsenoside Rg3 with docetaxel enhances the susceptibility of prostate cancer cells via inhibition of NF-κB. *Eur J Pharmacol.* 631(1): 1–9.

48. Yang, A.K., He, S.M., Liu, L., Liu, J.P., Wei, M.Q., and Zhou, S.F. (2010). Herbal interactions with anticancer drugs: mechanistic and clinical considerations. *Curr Med Chem.* 17: 1635–1678.

# PLANT MOLECULES

Phytochemicals are naturally occurring plant compounds such as glycosides, which is characterized by their strong foam-forming properties in aqueous solution. The concentration of active plant molecules varies among plant species. For example, saponins have been reported used in herbal medicine for treatment of diseases. There are about 150 kinds of natural saponins present in herbal medicine. Some of these saponins are reported to display anticancer activity *in vitro* and *in vivo* through varieties of signaling pathways associated with cell cycle.[1] In addition, there are saponins that remain to be characterized in details. The understanding of mechanism of action and structure–function relationships of saponins at the molecular and cellular levels provides insights into drug development.

## Aglycones

Aglycones have been reported to exhibit various biologic activities.[1-3] Aglycones are isoflavones that are present in soybean in two chemical forms, i.e., aglycones and glucosides. The difference in the absorption of soy isoflavone aglycones and glucosides in humans is attributed to the difference in chemical stucture.[3] After a single, low-dose intake (0.11 mmol), the highest isoflavone concentrations in plasma were reached 2 and 4 h after ingestion of aglycones and glucosides in humans. Subjects were four men (41-year-old) and four women (45-year-old). The highest plasma concentration after aglycone intake was more than two times greater than that after glucoside ingestion. In both high- and low-dose intake tests in human subjects, the plasma concentration of genistein was significantly higher than that of daidzein despite the similar levels of intake. After long-term (4-week) intakes (0.30 mmol/d), there was difference in plasma concentration of isoflavones (eight men, 45-year-old). After 2 and 4 weeks, these concentrations remained >100% higher after ingestion of aglycones than of glucosides. The results suggest that isoflavone aglycone-rich products may be more effective than glucoside-rich products in preventing chronic disease such as coronary heart disease. The anticancer effects of aglycones remain unclear.

## Ginsenosides

Ginsenosides belong to dammaranes and have been shown to inhibit tumor angiogenesis via suppressing development of endothelial cells of blood vessels and thereby preventing adhering, invasion, and metastasis of tumor cells.[1,2]

## Dioscin

One of the steroidal saponins and its aglycone diosgenin also has been extensively studied on its antitumor effect by cell cycle arrest and apoptosis.[1] Other important saponin molecules including avicins, platycodons, saikosaponins, and soysaponins along with tubeimosides were reported, but detail of the anticancer activity is lacking.

The incidence and treatment of cancer are a major worldwide health problem, with high endemicity in developing countries. In the absence of a satisfactory cancer drug, there is an urgent need for effective drugs and alternative medicine to replace or supplement those in current use. Traditional Chinese Medicine (TCM) is undoubtedly valuable source of new medicinal agents. The plant extracts and chemically defined molecules of natural origin showing anticancer activity are referred to a number of plant and herbal species and the parts utilized. The anticancer activity of recent TCM research on natural products is discussed.

The treatment strategy of cancer needs to be personalized because of individualized need and drug resistance. Metastasis of cancer remains a major challenge in treatment of cancer. Cancer patients present an immune deficiency and are not able to tolerate the side effects of drugs through a natural mechanism of defence. Moreover, cancer complications with diseases such as disorders of liver and kidney reduce the drug effects. Consequently, the complications increase the fatality of cancer patients if it is not diagnosed and treated in time. Although the problem of cancer therapy has been improved by the evolution of new cancer drugs, side effects and drug resistance present a limitation in drug use. Therefore, effective cancer therapy strategy with drugs in combination with TCM to supplement those in current use is an alternative approach to cancer therapy. The toxicity of clinically used drugs and the persistence of side effects even after modification of the dose level and duration of treatment is, however, severe drawbacks. The search for alternative cancer treatment strategy with novel agents is needed. Drugs coupled with TCM especially active natural products show promise.

In contrast, TCM extracts or plant-derived compounds are likely to provide a valuable source of novel agents.[3,4] The need for alternative treatment strategy has prompted the development of programs to screen natural products from TCM for the combination therapy of cancer.

In fact, the World Health Organization advocated the use of TCM where appropriate health services are not available.[4,5] Furthermore, the leads obtained from the search for natural products with anticancer activity prompt new impetus for obtaining valuable synthetic compounds.[6] Recent search on the use of natural products including plant extracts showed that active fractions and chemically defined molecules contained a small number of novel natural products and can be isolated and characterized.

## Anticancer activity of plant extracts and fractions

A TCM screening test for anticancer compounds was initiated in 1970 in China, based on the ethno-medical knowledge of the local population. The anticancer activity of plant extracts was evaluated *in vitro* and *in vivo* using animal models.[7] A number of herbs used topically in folk medicine in China and Asian countries to treat cancer were reported. Two plants were showed an *in vitro* antileishmanial activity: *Bocconia integrifolia* and *Begonia pearcei*. Three other plants, *Ampelocera edentula*, *Galipea longiflora*, and *Pera benensis*, employed by Chimane Indians, were effective in mice infected with *Leishmania amazonesis*.[8] However, these aqueous plant extracts did not show anticancer activity while the crude methanol extracts of other plant species revealed that the detail information of *in vitro* study with antileishmannial on pro-mastigotes was lacking.[4,9] However, the plant-based study did not show anticancer. Nevertheless, the potent anticancer activities of chemically defined molecules isolated from TCM origins could represent an exciting advance in the search for novel agents when there is a need for new drug development.

## An ayurvedic medicinal plant with anticancer activity

*Saussurea costus* (Falc.) Lipschitz, syn *Saussurea lappa* C.B. Clarke is a common medicinal plant used for the treatment of various ailments, namely asthma, inflammatory diseases, ulcer, and stomach problems. Sesquiterpene lactones have been reported as the major phyto-constituents of this species.[10,11]

S. *costus* exhibits anti-inflammatory, anti-ulcer, anticancer, and hepato-protective activities. Costunolide, dehydrocostus lactone (DL), and cynaropicrin, which were isolated from this plant, have been reported as bioactive molecules.[10] However, the detail of the anticancer activity of S. *costus* and its constituents is lacking. It is worth further investigating the chemistry, pharmacology, and folkloric uses of S. *costus*.

## Active compounds from *S. costus*

Costunolide, an active compound isolated from the root of S. *costus*, was reported to exhibit its effect on the induction of apoptosis in HL-60 human leukemia cells and its putative pathways of action.[11] Costunolide was reported to be able to induce apoptotic activity through modulating reactive oxygne species (ROS) generation, thereby resulting in mitochondrial permeability transition (MPT) and cytochrome *c* release to the cytosol was reduced. The apoptotic activities in costunolide-treated cells were shown to be inhibited by the antioxidant *N*-acetylcysteine (NAC). Cyclosporine A, a permeability transition inhibitor, was also shown to inhibit MPT and apoptosis. The results suggested that costunolide can be a good anticancer agent for drug development. This is the first report of the mechanism of the anticancer effect of constunolide.[11]

A previous study also reported the antitumor effects of S. *costus* on proliferation and expression of proteins associated with cell growth and apoptosis using an adenocarcinoma cells persistently infected with parainfluenza virus type 5 (PIV5).(ATCC® CRL-1739™); (AGS) gastric cancer cell line.[12,13] The study shown that *S. costus* reduced cell viabilities in a dose and time-dependent manner. *S. lappa* was shown to induce apoptotic cell death of AGS. Expression of gene product analyses by Reverse_transcription_polymerase_chain_reaction (RT-PCR) and Western blots revealed that it increased expression of the p53 and its downstream effector p21Waf1 and increased expression of apoptosis-related Bax and cleavage of active caspase-3 protein. The results indicated that *S. costus* induced cell growth inhibition and apoptosis of human gastric cancer cells, which are believed to be associated with downregulation and upregulation of cell growth regulating apoptotic and tumor suppressor genes.[13]

## The cytostatic effects of *S. costus* root

The cytostatic activities of *S. costus* root extract were attributed to the regulation of cyclins and pro-apoptotic intermediates and suppression of anti-apoptotic activities. The extracts of *S. costus* root with anticancer activity were used for the treatment of gastric cancers by combination therapy with cancer drugs.[12]

## Lappadilactone and seven sesquiterpene lactones

Sesquiterpene lactones of *S. costus* were shown to exhibit anticancer activity against selected human cancer cell lines.[14] Lappadilactone, DL, and costunolide exhibited the most potent cytotoxicity with CD50 values ranging from 1.6 to 3.5 g/mL in a dose- and time-dependent manner. The cytotoxicity showed similar activities against HepG2, OVCAR-3, and HeLa cell lines. The structure–activity relationship showed that the methylene-lactone moiety is involved for cytotoxic activity.

## DL, the major sesquiterpene lactone

DL was isolated from the roots of *S. costus*, which inhibited NF-kappa B activation through inhibition of tumor necrosis factor α (TNF-α) induced degradation and phosphorylation of its inhibitory protein I-kappa B alpha in human leukemia HL-60 cells. The results suggested that DL induced apoptosis via caspase-8 and caspase-3 activities.[15]

## Cynaropicrin, isolated from *S. lappa*

Cynaropicrin exhibited immunomodulating activity leading to cytokine release, nitric oxide production, and immunosuppressive effects. Cynaropicrin was shown to inhibit the proliferation of leukocyte cancer cell lines, such as U937, Eol-1, and Jurkat T cells, but Chang liver cells and human fibroblast cell lines were not inhibited to the same extent by cynaropicrin treatment. In contrast, the combination treatment with cysteine and NAC, reactive oxygen species scavengers, or rottlerin (1-[6-[(3-acetyl-2, 4, 6-trihydroxy-5-methylphenyl)methyl]-5,7-dihydroxy-2, 2-dimethyl-2*H*-1-benzopyran-8-yl]-3-phenyl-2-propen-1-one), a specific protein kinase (PK)C inhibitor, reduced cynaropicrin-mediated cytotoxicity and morphological change, and that cynaropicrin-induced proteolytic cleavage of PKC suggests that reactive oxygen species and PKC may play an important role in mediating pro-apoptotic activity by cynaropicrin. The results suggest that cynaropicrin is a good anticancer agent against some leukocyte cancer cells such as lymphoma or leukemia.[10,16]

## Costunolide, a sesquiterpene lactone isolated from *S. lappa*

Costunolide exhibited anticancer activity through an anti-angiogenic effect. This compound mediated vascular endothelial growth factor (VEGF), thereby inhibiting endothelial cell proliferation. It was also found to inhibit the VEGF-induced chemotaxis of human umbilical vein endothelial cells (HUVECs).[16] VEGF interacts with its cognate receptors, KDR/Flk-1 and Flt-1. The result showed that costunolide exerted inhibitory effects on angiogenesis by blocking the angiogenic factor signaling pathway. Costunolide also inhibited the autophosphorylation of KDR/Flk-1 without affecting that of Flt-1. These results suggest that costunolide was a novel inhibitor of angiogenesis.[17–19]

## C-17 polyene alcohol isolated from *S. costus*

C-17 polyene alcohol exhibited moderate cytotoxicities against the human tumor cell lines A549, SK-OV3, SK-MEL-2, XF 498, and HCT 15.[18] However, detail of the active components and anticancer activity remains unknown.

# Plant molecules with medicinal properties

Table 2.1 shows the common naturally occurring plant molecules with medicinal properties. A salient review of natural products with multi-arrays of biologic activity including anti-inflammatory, antileishmanial, anticancer, and immunomodulatory activity is included. However, details of anticancer activity of the common naturally occurring plant molecules remain unclear. Although individual phytochemicals display good *in vitro* and *in vivo*, test with animal models may show otherwise due to differences in hormonal control and physiological response between humans and the animal models. Therefore, a potential drug development based on naturally occurring molecules often met with disappointment. However, derivatization of various analogs would be helpful in the novel drug design especially with computer-aided design of analogs. Yet there are numerous hurdles to be overcome along the way in order to come up with an effective drug. Mass production and purity of the desirable products are crucial in novel drug development. Although a large number of plant molecules have been reported in the literature, not all of the molecules can exhibit biological activity in *in vivo* study. Within the fields of pharmacology and drug development, a plant molecule with a low molecular weight (<900 daltons) can be a better candidate to facilitate molecular interaction, specificity, and bioavailability in the body. Small plant organic compounds may regulate a biological process, with a size on the order of 1 nm (Appendix I). Most drugs are preferable small molecules.

**Table 2.1**  Small plant molecules with medicinal properties

| Compound | Source | Biological Activity | Reference |
|---|---|---|---|
| Picroliv | Root and rhizome of *Picrorhiza Kurroa* | • Hepatoprotective activity<br>• Significant antile-ishmanial activity | Rocha *et al.*[10] |
| Isotetrandrine | *Caulis Mahoniae* | • Antileishmanial activity | Rocha *et al.*[10] |
| Argentilactone | Roots of *Annona haematan-tha* | • Antileishmanial activity | Rocha *et al.*[10] |

| Compound | Source | Biological Activity | Reference |
|---|---|---|---|
| Luteolin | *Terminalia chebula* | • Anti-inflammation<br>• Inhibition of production of TNF-α<br>• Attenuation of ovalbumin-induced airway bronchoconstriction and bronchial hyperreactivity | Calixto *et al.*[20] |
| Nobiletin | Tangerine | • Anti-inflammation<br>• Immunomodulatory activity<br>• Antitumor activity | Calixto *et al.*[20] |
| Wogonin | *Scutellaria baicalensis* Georgi. | • Anti-inflammation: Treatment of bronchitis, nephritis, hepatitis, asthma, and atopic dermatitis | Calixto *et al.*[20] |
| Paeonol | *Paeonia suffruticosa, Arisaema erubescens, Dioscorea japonica* | • Analgesic and anti-inflammatory activity | Calixto *et al.*[20] |
| Glycyrrhetinic acid | *Glycyrrhiza glabra* (liquorice root) | • Improve the resistance to opportunistic infection of HSV-1, through induction of CD4+ T cells | Khan *et al.*[21] |

*(Continued)*

**Table 2.1** Small plant molecules with medicinal properties (*Continued*)

| Compound | Source | Biological Activity | Reference |
|---|---|---|---|
| Eugenol | Clove oil, nutmeg, cinnamon, basil, and bay leaf | • Provide significant protection against genital HSV-2 infection | Khan *et al.*[21] |
| Caffeic acid | Bark of *Eucalyptus globulus*, *Salvinia molesta*, *Phellinus linteus* | • Antiviral activity against HSV-1 | Khan *et al.*[21] |
| Dehydroxy-rooperol I and dehydroxy-rooperol II | Phenolic pent-4-en-1-yne derivatives | • Antiradical properties (antioxidant) | Kabanda *et al.*[22] |
| Rooperol | *Hypoxidaceae* spp. | • Antioxidant | Kabanda *et al.*[22], Boukes and van de Venter[23] |
| (-)-Epicatechin | *Geranium mexicanum* HBK. | • Antiamebic effect | Bolanos *et al.*[24] |
| Sulphoraphane | Isothiocyanate derived from cruciferous vegetables | • Mimic chemotherapeutic drugs | Ullah *et al.*[25] |
| Pomiferin | Isoflavonoid from *Maclura pomifera* | • Histone diacetylase inhibition activity | Ullah *et al.*[25] |

| Compound | Source | Biological Activity | Reference |
|---|---|---|---|
| Anacardic acid (6-penta-decylsalicylic acid) | Cashew nuts | • Anticancer, anti-inflammatory, and radiosensitization activities | Sung *et al.*[26] |
| Ginsenosides (dammaranes) | *Panax* (ginseng). | • Beneficial targeted on inhibition of tumor angiogenesis<br>• Prevention of adhering, invasion, and metastasis of tumor cells | Man *et al.*[1] |
| Dioscin | | • Antitumor effect by cell cycle arrest and apoptosis<br>• Protective effect against acetaminophen-induced liver damage | Man *et al.*[1], Zhao *et al.*[27] |
| Harmine | *Peganum harmala* | • Anticancer activity | Chen *et al.*[28] |
| Sesquiterpene lactones | *S. costus* | • Anti-inflammatory, anti-ulcer, anti-cancer, and hepatoprotective activities | Pandey *et al.*[11] |
| Theophylline | Green tea (*Camellia sinensis* L.) | • Antioxidant<br>• Treatment of respiratory diseases such as asthma | Sharangi[29] |

*(Continued)*

**Table 2.1** Small plant molecules with medicinal properties (*Continued*)

| Compound | Source | Biological Activity | Reference |
|---|---|---|---|
| Gallic acid | Bitter gourd (*Momordica charantia* L.) | • Antioxidant | Kubola and Siriamornpun[30] |
| Phelligridins D | *Inonotus obliquus* | • Anticancer | Lee *et al.*[31] |
| Diosgenin | Tubers of Dioscorea wild yam (Kokoro) | • Reduce the risk of cardiovascular diseases and aid in cardioprotection | Vasanthi *et al.*[32] |
| Tocotrienols | Vegetable oils, including rice bran oil and palm oil | • Cardioprotective effect | Vasanthi *et al.*[32] |
| Aloesin | *Aloe barbadensis* Mill. | • Radical scavenging activity → antioxidant | Lucini *et al.*[33] |
| Glucobrassicin (GBS) | Canescens flower buds | • Antioxidant and chemopreventive properties | Galletti *et al.*[34] |
| Scopoletin | *Rosa heckeliana* Tratt. roots | • Bacteriostatic activity<br>• Anti-inflammatory activity | Coruh and Ozdogan[35] |
| Verbascoside | Lamiales order (syn. Scrophulariales) | • Antioxidant | D'Imperio *et al.*[36] |

| Compound | Source | Biological Activity | Reference |
|----------|--------|---------------------|-----------|
| Ferulic acid | *Carpobrotus edulis, Ferula communis* | • Highest inhibitory activity against deoxyribose degradation | Soobrattee *et al.*[37] |
| Rosmarinic acid | *Lamiaceae* | • Antioxidant | Soobrattee *et al.*[37] |
| Gambierol | *Gambierdiscus toxicus* | • Antagonist of neurotoxin site 5 on neuronal voltage-gated sodium channels (VGSCs) | LePage *et al.*[38] |
| Pomolic acid | *Rosa woodsii, Euscaphis japonica, Uapaca togoensis* | • Anticancer properties through the modulation of activated protein kinase (AMPK) pathway plays a key role as a master regulator of cellular energy homeostasis | Youn *et al.*[39], Kuete *et al.*[40] |

# References

1. Man, S., Gao, W., Zhang, Y., Huang, L., and Liu, C. (2010). Chemical study and medical application of saponins as anti-cancer agents. *Fitoterapia.* 81: 703–714.
2. Wang, W., Zhao, Y., and Rayburn, E.R. (2007). In vitro anti-cancer activity and structure–activity relationships of natural products isolated from fruits of Panax ginseng. *Cancer Chemother Pharmacol.* 59: 589–601.
3. Izumi, T., Piskula, M.K., Osawa, S., *et al.* (2000). Soy isoflavone aglycones are absorbed faster and in higher amounts than their glucosides in humans. *J Nutr.* 130(7): 1695–1699.
4. Kayser, O., and Kiderlen, A.F. (2001). In vitro leishmanicidal activity of naturally occurring chalcones. *Phytother Res.* 15: 148–152.
5. Tahir, A.E., Ibrahim, A.M., Satti, G.M.H., Theander, T.G., Kharazmi, A., and Khslid, A.S. (1998). The potential antileishmanial activity of some Sudanese medicinal plants. *Phytother Res.* 12: 576–579.

6. Weniger, B., Robledo, S., Arango, G.J., *et al.* (2001). Antiprotozoal activities of Colombian plants. *J. Ethnopharmacol.* 78: 193–200.

7. Carvalho, P.B., Arribas, M.A.G., and Ferreira, E.I. (2000). Leishmaniasis. What do we know about its chemotherapy? *Rev Bras Ci Farm.* 36 (Suppl 1): 69–96.

8. Sauvain, M., Dedet, J.P., Kunesch, N., and Poisson, J. (1994). Isolation of flavans from the Amazonian shrub *Faramea guianensis. J Nat Prod.* 57: 403–406.

9. Fournet, A., Barrios, A.A., and Munoz, V. (1994). Leishmanicidal and trypanocidal activities of Bolivian medicinal plants. *J Ethnopharmacol.* 41: 19–37.

10. Rocha, L.G., Almeida, J.R.G.S., Macêdo, R.O., and Barbosa-Filho, J.M. (2005). A review of natural products with antileishmanial activity. *Phytomedicine.* 12: 514–535.

11. Pandey, M.M., Rastogi, S., and Rawat, A.K.S. (2007). *Saussurea costus*: botanical, chemical and pharmacological review of an ayurvedic medicinal plant. *J Ethnopharmacol.* 110: 379–390.

12. Lee, M.G., Lee, K.T., Chi, S.G., and Park, J.H. (2001). Costunolide induces apoptosis by ROS-mediated mitochondrial permeability and cytochrome C release. *Biol Pharm Bull.* 24: 303–306.

13. Ko, S.G., Kim, H.P., Jin, D.H., *et al.* (2005). *Saussurea lappa* induces G2-growth arrest and apoptosis in AGS gastric cancer cells. *Cancer Lett.* 220: 11–19.

14. Ko, S.G., Koh, S.H., Jun, C.Y., Nam, C.G., Bae, H.S., and Shin, M.K. (2004). Induction of apoptosis by *Saussurea lappa* and *Pharbitis nil* on AGS gastric cancer cells. *Biol Pharm Bull.* 27: 1604–1610.

15. Sun, C.M., Syu, W.J., Don, M.J., Lu, J.J., and Lee, G.H. (2003). Cytotoxic sesquiterpene lactones from the root of *Saussurea lappa. J Nat Prod.* 66: 1175–1180.

16. Oh, G.S., Pae, H.O., Chung, H.T., *et al.* (2004). Dehydrocostus lactone enhances tumor necrosis factor-alpha-induced apoptosis of human leukemia HL-60 cells. *Immunopharmacol Immunotoxicol.* 26: 163–175.

17. Cho, J.Y., Kim, A.R., Jung, J.H., Chun, T., Rhee, M.H., and Yoo, E.S. (2004). Cytotoxic and pro-apoptotic activities of cynaropicrin, a sesquiterpene lactone, on the viability of leukocyte cancer cell lines. *Eur J Pharmacol.* 92: 85–94.

18. Jeong, S.J., Itokawa, T., Shibuya, M., *et al.* (2002). Costunolide, a serquiterpene lactone from *Saussurea lappa* inhibits the VEGER KDR/FLK-1 signaling pathway. *Cancer Lett.* 187: 129–133.

19. Jung, I.H., Kim, Y., Lee, C., Kang, S.S., Park, J.H., and Im, K.S. (1998). Cytotoxic constituents of *Saussurea lappa. Arch Pharmacol Res.* 21: 153–156.

20. Calixto, J.B., Campos, M.M., Otuki, M.F., and Santos, A.R.S. (2004). Anti-inflammatory compounds of plant origin. Part II. Modulation of pro-inflammatory cytokines, chemokines and adhesion molecules. *Planta Med.* 70(2): 93–103.

21. Khan, M.T., Ather, A., Thompson, K.D., and Gambarim, R. (2005). Extracts and molecules from medicinal plants against herpes simplex viruses. *Antiviral Res.* 67(2): 107–119.

22. Kabanda, M.M., Mammino, L., Murulana, L.C., Mwangi, H.M., and Mabusela, W.T. (2015). Antioxidant radical scavenging properties of phenolic pent-4-en-1-yne derivatives isolated from *Hypoxis rooperi*. A DFT study in vacuo and in solution. *Int J Food Prop.* 18: 149–164.

23. Boukes, G.J., and van de Venter, M. (2012). Rooperol as an antioxidant and its role in the innate immune system: an in vitro study. *J Ethnopharmacol.* 144(3): 692–699.

24. Bolanos, V., Diaz-Martinez, A., Soto, J., *et al.* (2014). The flavonoid (-)-epicatechin affects cytoskeleton proteins and functions in *Entamoeba histolytica. J Proteomics.* 111: 74–85.

25. Ullah, M.F., Bhat, S.H., Husain, E., *et al.* (2014). Cancer chemopreventive pharmacology of phytochemicals derived from plants of dietary and non-dietary origin: implication for alternative and complementary approaches. *Phytochem Rev.* 13(4): 811–833.

26. Sung, B., Pandey, M.K., Ahn, K.S., *et al.* (2008). Anacardic acid (6-nonadecyl salicylic acid), an inhibitor of histone acetyltransferase, suppresses expression of nuclear factor-kappa B-regulated gene products involved in cell survival, proliferation, invasion, and inflammation through inhibition of the inhibitory subunit of nuclear factor-kappa B alpha kinase, leading to potentiation of apoptosis. *Blood.* 111(10): 4880–4891.

27. Zhao, X., Cong, X., Zheng, L., Xu, L., Yin, L., and Peng, J. (2012). Dioscin, a natural steroid saponin, shows remarkable protective effect against acetaminophen-induced liver damage in vitro and in vivo. *Toxicol Lett.* 214(1): 69–80.

28. Chen, Q., Chao, R.H., Chen, H.S., *et al.* (2005). Antitumor and neurotoxic effects of novel harmine derivatives and structure-activity relationship analysis. *Int J Cancer.* 114(5): 675–682.

29. Sharangi, A.B. (2009). Medicinal and therapeutic potentialities of tea (*Camellia sinensis* L.) — a review. *Food Res Int.* 42(5–6): 529–535.

30. Kubola, J., and Siriamornpun, S. (2008). Phenolic contents and antioxidant activities of bitter gourd (*Momordica charantia* L.) leaf, stem and fruit fraction extracts in vitro. *Food Chem.* 110(4): 881–890.

31. Lee, I.K., Kim, Y.S., Jang, Y.W., Jung, J.Y., and Yun, B.S. (2007). New antioxidant polyphenols from the medicinal mushroom *Inonotus obliquus. Bioorg Med Chem Lett.* 17(24): 6678–6681.

32. Vasanthi, H.R., ShriShriMal, N., and Das, D.K. (2012). Phytochemicals from plants to combat cardiovascular disease. *Curr Med Chem.* 19(14): 2242–2251.

33. Lucini, L., Pellizzoni, M., Pellegrino, R., Molinari, G.P., and Collam, G. (2015). Phytochemical constituents and in vitro radical scavenging activity of different Aloe species. *Food Chem.* 170: 501–507.

34. Galletti, S., Bagatta, M., Branca, F., *et al.* (2015). *Isatis canescens* is a rich source of glucobrassicin and other health-promoting compounds. *J Sci Food Agric.* 95(1): 158–164.

35. Coruh, N., and Ozdogan, N. (2015). Identification and quantification of phenolic components of *Rosa heckeliana* Tratt roots. *J Liq Chromatogr Rel Technol.* 38(5): 569–578.

36. D'Imperio, M., Cardinali, A., D'Antuono, I., *et al.* (2014). Stability-activity of verbascoside, a known antioxidant compound, at different pH conditions. *Food Res Int.* 66: 373–378.

37. Soobrattee, M.A., Neergheen, V.S., Luximon-Ramma, A., Aruoma, O.I., and Bahorun, T. (2005). Phenolics as potential antioxidant therapeutic agents: mechanism and actions. *Mutat Res.* 579(1–2): 200–213.

38. LePage, K.T., Rainier, J.D., Johnson, H.W., Baden, D.G., and Murray, T.F. (2007). Gambierol acts as a functional antagonist of neurotoxin site 5 on voltage-gated sodium channels in cerebellar granule neurons. *J Pharmacol Exp Ther.* 323(1): 174–179.

39. Youn, S.H., Lee, J.S., Lee, M.S., *et al.* (2012). Anticancer properties of pomolic acid-induced AMP-activated protein kinase activation in MCF7 human breast cancer cells. *Biol Pharm Bull.* 35(1): 105–110.

40. Kuete, V., Sandjo, L.P., Seukep, J.A., *et al.* (2015). Cytotoxic compounds from the fruits of *Uapaca togoensis* towards multifactorial drug-resistant cancer cells. *Planta Med.* 81(1): 32–38.

# HERBAL MEDICINES

Although various treatment methods for cancer therapy are available, drug treatment causes side effects that pose a limitation to cancer therapy. The drug cytotoxicity causes significant psychological and spiritual stress in cancer patients. Neither herbal medicines nor Western medicine alone can satisfactorily alleviate the stress associated with therapeutic drugs. Traditional Chinese Medicine (TCM) modalities offer less toxicity yet effective treatment for advanced cancers remains to be investigated. A combination of Western medicine and herbal medicines would complement each other for the treatment of cancer. Health risks of integrating herbal medicines with cancer drugs can be ameliorated. An integrative approach can harness the strength of Western medicine and herbal medicines.[1]

Cancer and the related complications significantly compromise body functions and affect the quality of life. The pharmacological effects of TCM as anticancer agents or as adjuvants can increase the cancer drug efficacy and ameliorate undesirable side effects of cancer drugs. The combination of drugs and TCM revealed that the anti-tumor immunity can be improved.[2]

## Herbal medicines as a rich source for drug development

Herbal medicine has become a rich source of anticancer agents and facilitated the development of cancer drugs. However, extensive screening tests of the potential active phytochemicals *in vitro* are needed. Effects of *in vitro* combination and characterization of potential anticancer phyto-chemicals against human cancer cell lines are studied. Effects of combi-nation of beta-elemene with taxanes were studied in human lung cancer cells.[3] Synergistic interactions were observed with combinations of ss-elemene and taxanes. This is related to the enhanced cytotoxicity of tax-anes via induction of cytochrome *c* release from mitochondria, caspase-8 and -3 cleavage, and down-regulation of Bcl-2 and Bcl-X-L expression. The anticancer activity of the combination of TCM and cancer drugs has raised tremendous interest worldwide.

## The health benefits of herbal medicine

The health benefits of herbal medicines are believed to be attributed to the interactions with anticancer compounds. This combination strategy for treatment of cancer is used to evaluate the composition of TCM for-mulation. Yanhusuo San consists of Rhizoma Corydalis and Rhizoma Curcumae was an ancient Chinese medicine prescription for treatment of cancer dated back in 960–1279 AD.[4] The common approach is to compare the $IC_{50}$ of each herbal extract and both extracts at different compositions by 3-(4,5-dimethylthiazol-2-yl)-2,5-diphenyl tetrazolium bromide (MTT) assay. The isobologram and combination index (CI) are used to evaluate the synergistic effects of the herbal extracts. Flow cytom-etry, fluorescence analysis, Western blot analysis, and gene expression profile can be used to fathom out the mechanism of actions of the herbal extracts. A plausible molecular mechanism of the synergistic anti-tumor effects of Rhizoma Corydalis and Rhizoma Curcumae was reported.[5]

## Activity-based fractionation of TCM extracts

The active fractions are derived from activity-based fractionation of herbal extracts *in vitro* and *in vivo* study. However, the anti-tumor activity of indi-vidual phytochemical may not show effects in animal study. Nevertheless, the composition of phytochemicals with anti-tumor effects in cancer cell lines can be evaluated *in vivo*. *Curcuma aromatica* and *Polygonum cuspida-tum* are one of the widely used herbs for liver cancer therapy. Curcumin, the active principle of *C. aromatica*, and resveratrol, the active principle of *P. cuspidatum*, contribute to the anticancer effects in colon cancer.[6] The combination of curcumin and resveratrol significantly inhibited the proliferation of Hepa-1-6 cells. The combination of phytochemicals may enhance the efficacy of herbal medicine. The combination of curcumin and reveratrol is a good example of an integrated method for liver cancer treatment.

## Use of bioinformatics

Current data basis of herbal medicine is limited. Bioinformatics on the selection and synergism of herbal extracts and constituents with anticancer properties are warranted to be developed. Chemo-informatics methodology can play an important role in clinical applications and are helpful in drug development. Novel herbal extract in combination of cancer drugs was characterized in ACHN and A2780/cp cells with chemo-bioinformatics-aided analysis.[7] Chemo-bioinformatics confirmed the predicted outcomes. The information could provide useful information on the use of herbs in reversing multidrug resistance (MDR).

## TCM as ingredients for food supplements

Herbal medicines are commonly used in food supplement for improving general health. Diet is not the primary therapy for refractory forms of cancer. Yet an appropriate food supplement may be effective as an adjuvant to hormone deprivation therapy for cancer. This treatment strategy could delay relapse and inhibit refractory growth. Zyflamend, a combination of multiple herbal extracts, was reported to exhibit anticancer properties.[8,9] Zyflamend can inhibit growth of various prostate cancer cell lines and androgen-dependent tumor growth in a mouse model at the advanced stages of prostate cancer. Herbal extracts as adjuvant in food supplements have become a common approach in cancer therapy. The active herbal extracts also exhibit chemo-protective properties against carcinogenesis.

## Effects of herbal formulations

Herbal medicines generally show health benefits toward different types of cancer, yet individual herbs do not display considerably activity. Herbal formulations coupled with drugs have been used as complementary and alternative medicine for cancer therapy. Although herbal medicines may take a longer period to show pharmacological effects in cancer patients, the adverse side effects of herbal medicines are minimal. Often, herbal formulations are preferred based on clinical practices. Teng-Long-Bu-Zhong-Tang (TLBZT) was demonstrated to show anticancer effects on colorectal cancer *in vitro*.[10–12] TLBZT significantly inhibited CT26 colon carcinoma growth via apoptotic caspase cascade. It can enhance the anticancer effects of 5-Fu in CT26 colon carcinoma.[12]

Herbal medicines are known to be able to enhance the efficacy of cancer drugs. A combination of the active constituents can be more effective anticancer agents. A combination of jaceosidin, emodin, and magnolol showed remarkable anticancer activities in melanoma A375.[11–13] The combination of these phytochemicals induced cell cycle arrest and consequently apoptosis in melanoma A375 cell line. However, a different combination of emodin with magnolol was more effective than the other combinations.

## Traditional herbal formulations

Traditional herbal formulations represent specific composition of herbal extracts prepared in boiling water. However, it is realized that high temperature of boiling may have a significant impact on the stability of phytochemicals.[12,13] The chemical properties of chlorogenic acid, an active component in green tea and TCM, can be changed through boiling yet the anticancer properties of chlorogenic acid and its derivatives remained the same against $CCl_4$-induced toxicity in hepG2 cells.[12,14] Herbal extraction of *Scutellaria baicalensis* Georgi, *Glycyrrhiza uralensis* Fisch, *Paeonia lactiflora* Pall, and *Ziziphus jujuba* Mill in boiling water would enhance the anticancer activities of chemotherapy in various cancers using various mouse tumor xenograft and allograft models.[13–15]

## Clinical evaluation of herbal medicines

Laboratory studies of herbal medicines are expanding the clinical knowledge. Different herbal extracts can be prepared as natural health products. Specific formulations are more effective to modulate angiogenesis and epidermal growth factor receptor and the related signaling pathways, which play a significant role in cancer growth. Quality assurance of specific herbal extracts is important as herbs obtained from different geographical regions might not have the same anticancer properties. Their effectiveness may be affected when multiple herbal agents are used. An integrative approach for managing cancer should target the multiple signaling pathways associated with cancer growth. Angiogenesis is an essential process in cancer development. Herbal products can affect angiogenesis and consequently inhibit cancer growth.[14] Herbal formulations were showed to exhibit anti-angiogenic activity. Examples of anti-angiogenic herbs include *Artemisia annua*, *Viscum album*, *Curcuma longa*, *S. baicalensis*, *Magnolia officinalis*, *Camellia sinensis*, *Ginkgo biloba*, *Panax ginseng*, and quercetin. Surprisingly, other active phytochemicals may not show high anticancer effects when used alone, yet they can interact with other components in the herbal extracts to produce anticancer activities. Baicalin, an active phytochemical with antipyretic properties, in combination with *Salvia miltorrhiza* or *C. sinensis* extracts showed anti-proliferation effects on the human breast cancer cell lines MCF-7 and T-47D.[15] The combination of active compounds from different classes offers either enhanced therapeutic benefits or anti-proliferative effects on tumor growth. The anti-proliferative effects of these compounds can be extended to other cancer types. The results suggest that these compounds in combination with herbal extracts may function through different mechanisms. The advantages of using herbal medicines in cancer therapy are demonstrated in different studies either in combination with cancer drugs or in combination with other herbal extracts.[10-15]

High failure rates with cancer chemotherapy, the high cost, and drug toxicity have prompted alternative approaches to cancer treatment and drug discovery. Common molecular basis of cancer biology has been discovered through advancements in genomics and proteomics. With the advent of biotechnologies, a large numbers of potential drug candidates can be tested against a particular molecular target; thus, novel cancer drugs derived from herbal principles can be developed. One of the most abundant natural source for active compounds is herbal medicines. Natural products and their derivatives have been purified and structurally identified from herbal medicines. These active phytochemicals exhibit immense pharmacological and anticancer properties. Although the molecular mechanism of actions of active anticancer phytochemicals are yet to be elucidated, extensive research in herbal medicine continues to generate new data that are worth investigated further in clinical testing. Recent advancement in biotechnology and chemical technology has enabled us to understand salient interactions of natural products and their derivatives with cancer cells. As a result, the findings allow us to better design cancer drugs. Both the natural products and synthetic molecules share high chemical selectivity and pharmacological specificity. The ability of novel natural products to interact with specific protein domains would trigger a chain of cellular signaling processes. By virtue of specific binding affinity to gene products natural products can provide effective scaffolds for the pharmacological processes.[16] Potent natural products can show properties specified in the "Lipinski's rule of five."[17] The application of bioinformatics to quality control and efficacy of natural product derivatives, in particular small natural molecules should be used to enhance the interactions with molecular targets. However, these small naturally occurring natural products may involve multiple cellular targets and pathways. The inhibition of multiple mechanistic pathways may ameliorate chemo-resistance in various cancers. A better understanding of the interactions between natural compounds and the derivatives in cancer cells is pivotal for development of targeted anticancer agents. The discovery and development of potent anticancer agents from herbal medicines are hampered by lack of preclinical model for evaluation of the potency of anticancer phytochemicals. However, xenograft models and transgenic models can serve as a surrogate role in developing therapeutic anticancer drugs. Nevertheless, these models can show significant biochemical and physiological difference in humans. One of the potential issues associated with animal models for evaluation of potential drug efficacy is inappropriate dosing. With the improvement of animal models for human tumors at different developing stages, anticancer activities of potent phytochemicals that are identified from herbal extracts are likely to be helpful in drug development.[18]

Identification of specific biomarkers in cancer therapeutics is essential for comparison of efficacy of potential phytochemicals from herbal extracts. Bioinformatics on different biological systems offers useful information related to molecular signaling activity and assays for cancer biomarkers.

The use of herbal formulation for cancer therapy lies in the documented ancient formula and the quality of herbs that can vary significantly in phytochemical contents and anticancer properties due to geographical difference in herbal medicines. This has hampered the clinical use of ancient herbal formulation for treatment of cancer. Establishment of a causal relationship between a potent anticancer photochemical and cancer remains a challenge. Although cancer biology has been helpful in fathoming out the pathogenesis, only a limited number of the preventive measures based on herbal medicines are successful in human. However, herbal medicines remain one of the rich resources of anticancer agents for novel drug development. A combination strategy with cancer drugs and herbal medicines should be established for cancer therapy.

## Tamaractam, a new bioactive lactam, from *Tamarix ramosissima* induces apoptosis

Recent study showed *Tamarix ramosissima* Ledeb., a traditional herbal medicine used for treatment of rheumatoid arthritis (RA) in northwest China, led to the discovery of a new phenolic aromatic rings substituted lactam, tamaractam (Figure 3.1).[19] Tamaractam showed inhibition of RA-fibroblast-like synoviocytes (RA-FLSs). The terminal deoxynucleotidyl transferase-mediated dUTP nick-end labeling (TUNEL) assay showed activation of caspase-3/7 level using luminescence assay and sub-$G_1$ fraction measurement using flow cytometry. It was found that tamaractam displayed variable proliferation inhibitory activity in RA-FLS. Tamaractam could remarkably induce cellular apoptosis of RA-FLS, increase activated caspase-3/7 levels, and significantly increase sub-$G_1$ fraction in the cell cycle. The results suggested that tamaractam induced apoptosis through caspase cascade.

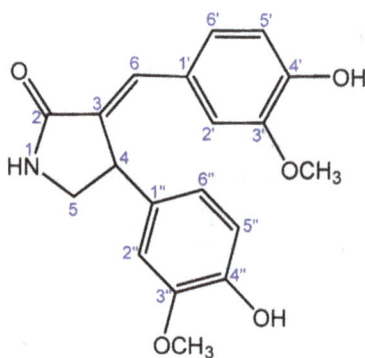

**Figure 3.1** Chemical structure of tamaractam.

(*E*)-3-(4'-Hydroxy-3'-methoxybenzylidene)-4-(4"-hydroxy-3"-methoxyphenyl) pyrrolidin-2-one (generically named tamaractam)

| | |
|---|---|
| Chemical formula | $C_{19}H_{19}NO_5$ |
| Molar mass | 342.13 g/mol |

- Tamaractam was isolated from *T. ramosissima*.
- Tamaractam was obtained as a white amorphous powder.
- Tamaractam has remarkable apoptosis-inducing effect on RA-FLS.

# Lucidumol C, a new cytotoxic lanostanoid triterpene, from *Ganoderma lingzhi* against human cancer cells

A new oxygenated lanostane-type triterpene, named lucidumol C was isolated from the chloroform extract of the fruiting bodies of *Ganoderma lingzhi*.[20] Structures were established based on Nuclear magnetic resonance (NMR) spectroscopic data. Potential cytotoxic activities of the isolated compound were shown to inhibit human colorectal carcinoma (HCT-116, Caco-2), human liver carcinoma (HepG2), and human cervical carcinoma (HeLa) cell lines using WST-1 reagent. Selectivity was evaluated using normal human fibroblast cells (TIG-1 and HF19). The result showed lucidumol C was potent selective cytotoxicity against HCT-116 cells with an $IC_{50}$ value of 7.86 ± 4.56 µM and selectivity index (SI) >10 with remarkable cytotoxic activities against Caco-2, HepG2, and HeLa cell lines.[20]

The following information summarized the biologic origin and anti-cancer activity of lucidumol C:

- Lucidumol C was isolated from the chloroform extract of the fruiting bodies of *G. lingzhi*.
- Lucidumol C is a new oxygenated lanostane-type triterpene.
- Lucidumol C has potent selective cytotoxicity against human colorectal carcinoma cells and remarkable cytotoxic activities against human colorectal carcinoma, human liver carcinoma, and human cervical carcinoma cell lines.

# Physcion-8-*O*-β-D-monoglucoside, a novel ligands for tumor necrosis factor-α and tumor necrosis factor receptor-1

Tumor necrosis factor-α (TNF-α) has been a validated therapeutic target for autoimmune diseases. All therapeutics used to target TNF-α are macromolecules, and limited numbers of TNF-α chemical inhibitors have been reported, which prompts the identification of small-molecule alternatives as needed. Recent studies with TCM have focused on identifying small molecules that directly bind to TNF-α or TNF receptor-1 (TNFR1) and to inhibit the interaction between TNF-α and TNFR1 with regulatory effects on related signaling pathways.[21-23] Recent study showed using pharmaco-phore model filtering and molecular docking was able to identify TNF-α antagonists. The residues in TNF-α that have been reported to play import-ant roles in the TNF-α–TNFR1 complex were removed in order to form a pocket for virtual screening of TNFR1-binding ligands. The results showed one ligand that could bind to TNFR1 and four ligands with different scaf-folds that bind to TNF-α. T1 and R1 with activities similar to those of known antagonists. The cell-based assays also demonstrated that T1 and R1 have similar activities compared with the known TNF-α antagonist C87. The results demonstrate that physcion-8-O-β-d-monoglucoside is a potent antagonist for TNF-α- and TNFR1-based drug development.[23]

The chemical structure of physcion-8-O-β-D-monoglucoside is shown in Figure 3.2 with biologic activity described below:

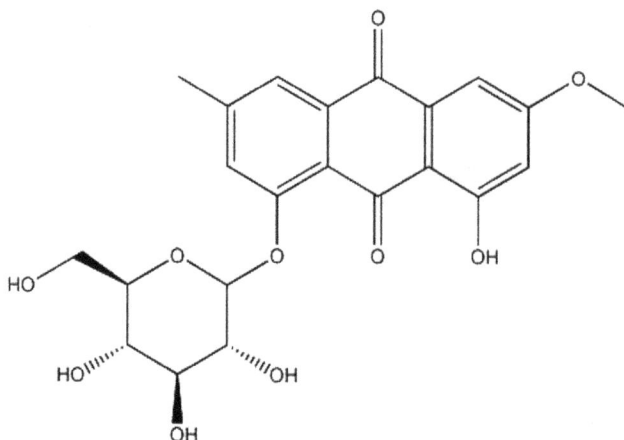

**Figure 3.2** The chemical structure of physcion-8-O-β-D-monoglucoside.

| Chemical formula | $C_{22}H_{22}O_{10}$ |
| --- | --- |
| Molar mass | 446.40408 g/mol |

- Physcion-8-O-β-D-monoglucoside is *Rheum officinale* extract.
- Physcion-8-O-β-D-monoglucoside was found for the first time that physcion-8-O-β-D-monoglucoside was a ligand for TNF receptor from herbal medicines.

- Pharmacological assays revealed that physcion-8-*O*-β-D-monoglucoside inhibited TNF-α-induced cytotoxicity and apoptosis in L929 cells via TNFR1.
- Although physcion-8-*O*-β-D-monoglucoside was a trace component in the chemical constituents of the *R. officinale* extract, it had considerable anti-inflammatory activities.[23]

# References

1. Yang, A.K., He, S.M., Liu, L., Liu, J.P., Wei, M.Q., and Zhou, S.F. (2010). Herbal interactions with anticancer drugs: mechanistic and clinical considerations. *Curr Med Chem.* 17: 1635–1678.
2. Engdal, S., Klepp, O., and Nilsen, O.G. (2009). Identification and exploration of herb-drug combinations used by cancer patients. *Integr Cancer Ther.* 8: 29–36.
3. Li, P., Chen, J., Wang, J., *et al.* (2014). Systems pharmacology strategies for drug discovery and combination with applications to cardiovascular diseases. *J Ethnopharmacol.* 151(1): 93–107.
4. Wang, H., Chan, Y.L., Li, T.L., and Wu, C.J. (2012). Improving cachectic symptoms and immune strength of tumor-bearing mice in chemotherapy by a combination of *Scutellaria baicalensis* and Qing-Shu-yi-Qi-Tang. *Eur J Cancer.* 48: 1074–1084.
5. Gao, J.L., He, T.C., Li, Y.B., and Wang, Y.T. (2009). A traditional Chinese medicine formulation consisting of Rhizoma Corydalis and Rhizoma Curcumae exerts synergistic anti-tumor activity. *Oncol Rep.* 22: 1077–1083.
6. Zhao, J., Li, Q.Q., Zou, B., *et al.* (2007). In vitro combination characterization of the new anticancer plant drug beta-elemene with taxanes against human lung carcinoma. *Int J Oncol.* 31: 241–252.
7. Lau, C., Mooiman, K.D., Maas-Bakker, R.F., Beijnen, J.H., Schellens, J.H., and Meijerman, I. (2013). Effect of Chinese herbs on CYP3A4 activity and expression in vitro. *J Ethnopharmacol.* 149: 543–549.
8. Du, Q., Hu, B., An, H.M., *et al.* (2013). Synergistic anticancer effects of curcumin and resveratrol in Hepal-6 hepatocellular carcinoma cells. *Oncol Rep.* 29: 1851–1858.
9. Ghavami, G., Sardari, S., and Shokrgozar, M.A. (2011). Cheminformatics-based selection and synergism of herbal extracts with anti-cancer agents on drug resistance tumor cells-ACHN and A2780/CP cell lines. *Comput Biol Med.* 41: 665–674.
10. Huang, E.C., McEntee, M.F., and Whelan, J. (2012). Zyflamend, a combination of herbal extracts, attenuates tumor growth in murins xenograft models of prostate cancer. *Nutr Cancer Int J.* 64: 749–760.
11. Park, K.W., Ye, S.H., Kim, Y.J., *et al.* (2010). In vitro and in vivo anti-tumor effects of oriental herbal mixtures. *Food Sci Biotechnol.* 19: 1019–1027.
12. Deng, S., Hu, B., An, H.M., *et al.* (2013). Teng-Long-Bu-Zhong-Tang, a Chinese herbal formula, enhances anticancer effects of 5-Fluorouracil in CT26 colon carcinoma. *BMC Complement Altern Med.* 13: 128–134.
13. Shawi, A., Kimatu, J.N., Khan, M., and Hussain, K.A. (2011). Enhancement of induced apoptosis in human melanoma A375 by a combination of natural compounds. *J Med Plants Res.* 5: 5400–5406.

14. Kan, S., Cheung, M.W.M., Zhou, Y., and Ho, W.S. (2013). Effects of boiling on chlorogenic acid and the liver protective effects of its main products against CCl4-induced toxicity in vitro. *J Food Sci.* 79(2): c147–c154.

15. Liu, S.H., and Cheng, Y.C. (2012). Old formula, new Rx: the journey of PHY906 as cancer adjuvant therapy. *J Ethnopharmacol.* 140: 614–623.

16. Sagar, S.M., Yance, D., and Wong, R.K. (2006). Natural health products that inhibit angiogenesis: a potential source for investigational new agents to treat cancer. *Curr Oncol.* 1: 14–26.

17. Franek, K.J., Zhou, Z., Zhang, W.D., and Chen, W.Y. (2005). In vitro studies of baicalin alone or in combination with *salvia miltiorrhiza* extract as a potential anti-cancer agent. *Int J Oncol.* 26: 217–224.

18. Peczuh, M.W., and Hamilton, A.D. (2000). Peptide and protein recognition by designed molecules. *Chem Rev.* 100: 2479–2494.

19. Yao, Y., Cheng-Shuai, J., Na, S., Li, W.Q., *et al.* (2017). Tamaractam, a new bioactive lactam from *Tamarix ramosissima*, induces apoptosis in rheumatoid arthritis fibroblast-like synoviocytes. *Molecules.* 96: 22–40.

20. Amen, Y.M., Zhu, Q., Tran, H.B., *et al.* (2016). Lucidumol C, a new cytotoxic lanostanoid triterpene from *Ganoderma lingzhi* against human cancer cells. *J Nat Med.* 70(3): 661–666.

21. Cao, Y., Li, Y.H., Ly, D.Y., *et al.* (2016). Identification of a ligand for tumor necrosis factor receptor from Chinese herbs by combination of surface plasmon resonance biosensor and UPLC-MS. *Anal Bioanal Chem.* 408(19): 5359–5367.

22. Wen, X., Luo, K., Xiao, S., Ai, N., Wang, S., and Fan, X. (2016). Qualitative analysis of chemical constituents in traditional Chinese medicine analogous formula cheng-Qi decoctions by liquid chromatography–mass spectrometry. *Biomed Chromatogr.* 30(3): 301–311.

23. Chen, S., Feng, Z., Wang, Y., *et al.* (2017). Discovery of novel ligands for TNF-α and TNF receptor-1 through structure-based virtual screening and biological assay. *J Chem Inf Model.* 57(5): 1101–1111.

# THERAPEUTIC USES OF SMALL MOLECULES

Natural polyphenols, such as resveratrol (Res), present in different plants and vegetables. Res exhibits potential therapeutic activity with cardioprotective, anti-neurodegenerative, antioxidant, and antitumor action. The effect of Res on the mutual interactions between positively charged poly-L-lysine (PLL) and negatively charged dipalmitoylphosphatidylcholine/dipalmitoylphosphatidylglycerol (DPPC/DPPG) membranes was studied using Fourier-transform infrared (FTIR) spectroscopy supported by principal component analysis (PCA).[1] The interactions between PLL and DPPC/DPPG membranes were strongly affected by the presence of Res molecules. The concentration of Res affected membrane-induced transition of PLL from α-helix to an extended left-handed polyproline II helix (PPII) and occurred at different temperatures, with different cooperativities. The influence of PLL on the conformational (trans/gauche) state of the hydrocarbon chain region of the lipid membranes was modulated by Res.

## *Houttuynia cordata* Thunb. (Family: Saururaceae), a common medicinal plant

*Houttuynia cordata* Thunb. (Family: Saururaceae) is an herbaceous perennial plant that is well known among Asians in Japan, Korea, China, and Northeast India for its medicinal properties. The plant extract is used for treatment of ailments against inflammation, pneumonia, severe acute respiratory syndrome, muscular sprain, stomach ulcer, and cancer-related complications.

Oxidative stress and inflammation were found to be linked with most of the diseases in recent times. Many ancient texts from Chinese Traditional Medicine, Ayurveda and Siddha, and Japanese Traditional medicine have documented the efficacy of *H. cordata* against oxidative stress and inflammation.[2]

Efficacy of *H. cordata* extracts and its bioactive compounds both *in vitro* and *in vivo*, against oxidative stress and inflammation, was reported.[2]

Herbal medicines or plant products can be used for ameliorating the oxidative stress and treatment of inflammation-related diseases. *H. cordata* is known to target several signaling pathways and found to effectively reduce the oxidative stress and inflammation. Phyto-constituents such as afzelin, hyperoside, and quercitrin have strong antioxidant properties to reduce inflammation both *in vitro* and *in vivo* models. No detail of the anticancer activity was known.

## The antioxidant from the root of *Arctotis arctotoides* (L.f.)

The antioxidant and antimicrobial activities of the acetone, methanol, and water extracts from the root of *Arctotis arctotoides* (L.f.) O. Hoffm (Asteraceae) were reported to exhibit significant activity against both Gram-positive and Gram-negative bacteria. The strongest activity was found in the acetone extract on *Bacillus cereus*, *Staphylococcus aureus*, *Micrococcus kristinae*, and *Streptococcus pyrogens* with an Minimum Inhibitory Concentration Test (MIC) of 0.1 mg/mL.[3] Although not completely fungicidal, these extracts showed significant growth inhibition against all the fungi tested. Antioxidant and antimicrobial activities of the extracts were strongly correlated with total phenols and to a lesser extent with their flavonoid and pro-anthocyanidin contents. The results have validated the medicinal potential of the underground part of *A. arctotoides*.[3] However, the detail of the composition of active ingredients of the root extracts is lacking. Nevertheless, the medicinal potential of the root of *A. arctotoides* has not been revealed.

# Anti-tumorigenic activity of chrysin from *Oroxylum indicum*

It is well known that the p53 tumor suppressor gene plays critical roles in cell cycle regulation and apoptotic cell death in response to various cellular stresses, thereby preventing cancer development. Therefore, a common approach to the activation of p53 is through small plant molecules that can be an attractive therapeutic strategy for the treatment of cancers. A library of 700 Myanmar wild plant extracts to identify small molecules that induce p53 transcriptional activity was reported.[4] A cell-based screening method with a p53-responsive luciferase reporter assay system revealed that an ethanol extract of *Oroxylum indicum* bark increased p53 transcriptional activity. Chrysin was isolated and identified as the active ingredient in the *O. indicum* bark extract. Chrysin was shown to increase p53 protein expression and the p53-mediated expression of downstream target genes and decreased cell viability in MCF7 cells, but not in p53-knockdown MCF7 cells. It was also found that chrysin activated the ATM–Chk2 pathway in the absence of DNA damage. The results suggest the potential of chrysin as an anticancer drug.

# Plant molecule as sources of recombinant anticancer agents

Herbal plants were the first medicines used by humans and in folk medicine due to the many pharmacologically active compounds present in plants. Some of these compounds can display profound inhibitory effects on cell division and can therefore be used for the treatment of cancer, e.g., the mitostatic drug paclitaxel (Taxol).[5] The potential of active compounds to produce medicines targeting cancer has expanded due to the advent of computer-aided design synthesis and genetic engineering particularly in recent years because of the development of gene editing systems such as the CRISPR/Cas9 platform. These technologies allow the introduction of genetic modifications that facilitate the production heterologous recombinant proteins, including human antibodies, lectins, and vaccine candidates. The anticancer agents that are produced by plants and genetic modification can be developed in healthcare products. However, proteinaceous anticancer agents are also available. The proteinaceous products can exhibit an improved selectivity and reduced side effects compared with small molecule-based drugs.

## Inhibitor of cyclin-dependent kinase-2

Cyclin-dependent kinase-2 (CDK2) is a member of serine/threonine protein kinase family. It plays an important role in regulation of various eukaryotic cell cycle activities. Inhibition of CDK2 overexpression during cell cycle may modulate several cellular functional aberrations in human cancers including lung cancer, primary colorectal carcinoma, ovarian cancer, melanoma, and pancreatic carcinoma.[6] Phytochemicals of medicinal plants have been used as anticancer agents. The potential of active compounds as an alternative drug resource is excellent. Recent study showed anticancer phytochemicals from medicinal plants were able to inhibit CDK2.[6] Molecular Operating Environment (MOE v2009) software was used to dock 2300 phytochemicals in the study. The screening study shows that four phytochemicals such as Kushenol T, Remangiflavanone B, Neocalyxins A, and Elenoside bind strongly with all eight active residues Tyr15, Lys33, Ileu52, Lys56, Leu78, phe80, Asp145, and Phe146 of CDK2-binding site. These phytochemicals inhibited the CDK2 can be considered as potential anticancer agents and used in drug development against CDK2. It is expected that the results would pave way for phytochemical-based novel small molecules as anticancer therapeutic compounds with specificity.

## Anticancer activity of constituents of *Glycyrrhiza uralensis* (licorice)

Traditional Chinese medicines are known to exhibit significant bioactivities in folk medicine for treatment of various ailments. A combined strategy using both phytochemical and biological approaches was useful to discern the effective components of licorice, which is one of the most common herbs used in China. Altogether, 122 compounds (1–122), including six new structures (1–6), were isolated and identified from the roots and rhizomes of *Glycyrrhiza uralensis* (licorice). These compounds were assay-based test using 11 cell- and enzyme-based bioassay methods, including nuclear factor erythroid 2-related factor 2 (Nrf2) activation, NO inhibition, NF-κB inhibition, H1N1 virus inhibition, cytotoxicity for cancer cells (HepG2, SW480, A549, MCF7), PTP1B inhibition, tyrosinase inhibition, and

Acetylcholinesterase (AChE) inhibition. A number of bioactive compounds, particularly isoprenylated phenolics, were found for the first time.[7] Echinatin (7), a potent Nrf2 activator, attenuated $CCl_4$-induced liver damage in mice (5 or 10 mg/kg, ip) and thus is believed to be responsible for the hepato-protective activity of licorice (Figure 4.1).[7]

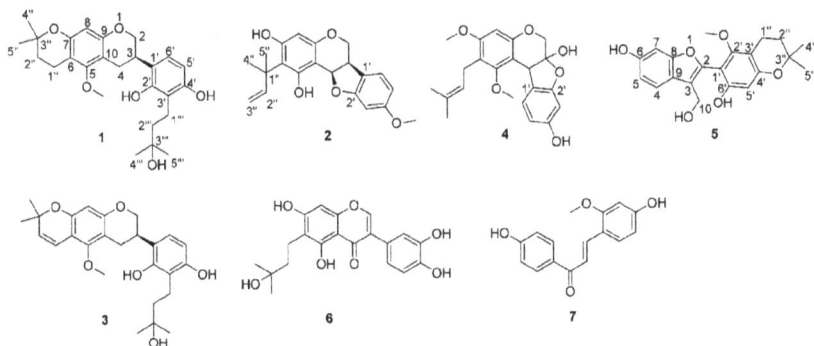

**Figure 4.1** Structures of compounds 1–7.

Stress can be caused by food metabolism and disturbances in hormone. Oxidative stress can cause various diseases and imbalance of body functions including kidney and liver disorders, chronic inflammation, and cancer.[8] Previous study has indicated that licorice shows hepato-protective and anti-cancer and antioxidative activities.[9,10] Nrf2 is a redox-sensitive transcription factor, which binds to antioxidant response elements (AREs) located in the promoter region of genes encoding antioxidant enzymes such as heme oxygenase-1 (HO-1) and glutathione (GSH) peroxidase (GPx).[11] An earlier study demonstrated the activation of the licorice compounds using a luciferase reporter assay in HepG2 human hepatocellular carcinoma cells stably transfected with Nrf2 luciferase reporter (HepG2C8 cells).[12] However, various compounds of licorice were reported to show multi-arrays of biologic activities with different mechanistic actions of active compounds. Many mechanisms are involved in the protective effects of glycyrrhizic acid and 18β-glycyrrhetinic acid in the liver functions leading to reduction of Aspartate aminotransferase (AST), (also called glutamic oxaloacetic transaminase (GOT)) and alanine aminotransferase (ALT), (also called glutamic pyruvic transaminase (GPT)), activities. The pregnane X receptor (PXR), as well as the cytochrome P450 family 3 subfamily A (CYP3A), can also be modulated by glycyrrhizic acid to protect against lithocholic acid-induced injury.[13]

Both glycyrrhizic acid and 18β-glycyrrhetinic acid treatments can inhibit liver fibrosis, which is believed to cause cancer.[14]

# References

1. Cieslik-Boczula, K. (2018). Influence of resveratrol on interactions between negatively charged DPPC/DPPG membranes and positively charged poly-L-lysine. *Chem Phys Lipids.* 214: 24–34. doi: 10.1016/j.chemphyslip.2018.05.004

2. Shingnaisui, K., Tapan, D., Prasenjit, M., and Jatin K. (2018). Therapeutic potentials of *Houttuynia cordata* Thunb. against inflammation and oxidative stress: a review. *J Ethnopharmacol.* 220: 35–43. doi: 10.1016/j.jep.2018.03.038

3. Afolayan, A.J., and Jimoh, F.O. (2009). Nutritional quality of some wild leafy vegetables in South Africa. *Int J Food Sci Nutr.* 60(5): 424–431. doi: 10.1080/09637480701777928

4. Nagasaka, M., Hashimoto, R., Inoue, Y., *et al.* (2018). Anti-tumorigenic activity of chrysin from *oroxylum indicum* via non-genotoxic p53 activation through the ATM-Chk2 pathway. *Molecules.* 23(6): 1394–1405. doi: 10.3390/molecules23061394

5. Buyel, J.F. (2018). Plants as sources of natural and recombinant anti-cancer agents. *Biotechnol Adv.* 36(2): 506–520. doi: 10.1016/j.biotechadv.2018.02.002

6. Khan, W., Ashfaq, U.A., Aslam, S., *et al.* (2017). Anticancer screening of medicinal plant phytochemicals against cyclin-dependent kinase-2: an in-silico approach. *Adv Life Sci.* 4(4): 113–119.

7. Shuai, J., Li, Z., and Song, W., *et al.* (2016). Bioactive constituents of *Glycyrrhiza uralensis* (Licorice): discovery of the effective components of a traditional herbal medicine. *J Nat Prod.* 79(2): 281–292. doi: 10.1021/acs.jnatprod.5b00877

8. Kensler, T.W., Wakabayashi, N., and Biswal, S. (2007). Cell survival responses to environmental stresses via the Keap1-Nrf2-ARE pathway. *Annu Rev Pharmacol Toxicol.* 47: 89–116. doi: 10.1146/annurev.pharmtox.46.120604.141046

9. Wang Z.Y., and Nixon D.W. (2001). Licorice and cancer. *J Nutr Cancer.* 39(1): 1–11. doi: 10.1207/S15327914nc391_1

10. Kao, T.C., Wu, C.H., and Yen, G.C. (2014). Bioactivity and potential health benefits of licorice. *J Agric Food Chem.* 62: 542–553. doi: 10.1021/jf404939f

11. Hwang, I.K., Lim, S.S., Choi, K.H., *et al.* (2006). Neuroprotective effects of roasted licorice, not raw form, on neuronal injury in gerbil hippocampus after transient forebrain ischemia. *Acta Pharmacol Sin.* 27: 959–965.

12. Gumpricht, E., Dahl, R., Devereaux, M.W., and Sokol, R.J. (2005). Licorice compounds glycyrrhizin and 18beta-glycyrrhetinic acid are potent modulators of bile acid-induced cytotoxicity in rat hepatocytes. *J Biol Chem.* 280: 10556–10563.

13. Wang, Y.G., Zhou, J.M., Ma, Z.C., *et al.* (2012). Pregnane X receptor mediated-transcription regulation of CYP3A by glycyrrhizin: a possible mechanism for its hepatoprotective property against lithocholic acid-induced injury. *Chem Biol Interact.* 200: 11–20.

14. Moro, T., Shimoyama, Y., Kushida, M., *et al.* (2008). Glycyrrhizin and its metabolite inhibit Smad3-mediated type I collagen gene transcription and suppress experimental murine liver fibrosis. *Life Sci.* 83: 531–539.

# MECHANISM OF ACTION

Apoptosis is a programmed cell death, which safeguards the organism by eliminating abnormal cells to maintain normal functions of the body. Apoptosis involves complex molecular events through activation of caspase cascade in cysteine and aspartic acid proteases. The activation of caspases is important in regulation of cell differentiation and death.

## Understanding of apoptotic activity

An understanding of signaling pathways with the cloning and characterization of pro- or anti-apoptotic genes has prompted the development of anticancer agents and herbal medicine for cancer therapy and diseases. Cell death may occur through either necrosis or apoptosis. Necrosis is a cell death in response to trauma generated by external factors or cell injury. Necrosis is characterized by swelling and rupture of the plasma cell membrane with the release of the cellular contents into the immediate extracellular space, which may cause inflammation to other neighboring cells.

In contrast to necrosis, apoptosis is a programmed cell death and regulated genetically and evolutionarily conserved form of cell death. Apoptosis is characterized by morphological and biochemical aspects including the condensation of the nucleus and cytoplasm and the activation of caspases and nucleases, which degrade cellular proteins and deoxyribonucleic acid (DNA), membrane blebbing, and the fragmentation of cells into multiple small membrane-bound apoptotic intermediates, which are rapidly phagocytosed by neighboring cells.[1-3] As a result, apoptotic cells are removed to regulate cell differentiation and growth. Deregulation of apoptosis may cause pathological conditions such as cancer or neurodegenerative diseases. Many important genes are responsible for the genesis of various cancers. The points of mutation were identified, and the related pathways were characterized. Understanding the complex interplay among apoptosis, autophagy, and necrosis may enable scientists and clinicians to reduce cancer development. Recent studies have contributed to the advancement of knowledge that facilitates better understanding of cancer initiation and progression with the three distinctive types of cell death including necrosis, apoptosis, and autophagy. A better understanding of the apoptotic signaling pathways may aid development of new targeted anticancer therapeutic strategies. The purposes of identification and characterization of anticancer agents from herbal medicine are to highlight examples of progress in these areas and to point out fertile grounds for future investigation.

## Molecular mechanism of programmed cell death and cancer

Cancer, a complex genetic disease, can develop from mutation of oncogenes or tumor suppressor genes. Abnormal cell growth can be developed due to alteration of signaling pathways.[1,4-5] Apoptosis occurs when DNA damage is irreparable.

Two core pathways exist to induce apoptosis, namely

- The extrinsic—death receptor (DR) pathway
- The intrinsic—mitochondrial pathway

The extrinsic pathway is triggered by binding of Fas plasma membrane DR and other similar receptors such as tumor necrosis receptor 1 and its relatives with its extracellular ligand, Fas-L. The Fas/Fas-L composite interacts with death domain-containing protein (Fas-associated death domain [FADD]) and pro-caspase-8, resulting to become the death-inducing signaling complex (DISC). Subsequently, the protein complex activates its pro-caspase-8, which proceeds to trigger pro-caspase-3, the enzyme responsible for execution of the apoptotic process.[6,7] The activation of intrinsic pathway also leads to apoptosis but under the control of mitochondrial pro-enzymes. Apoptosis can be initiated by either extracellular stimuli or intracellular signals. Outer mitochondrial membranes become permeable resulting in releasing of internal cytochrome *c* in the cytosol. Cytochrome *c* binds with apoptotic peptidase activating factor-1 (Apaf-1), and pro-caspase-9 to downstream triggers a caspase 9/3 signaling cascade, culminating in apoptosis.[8] Consequently, the initiation of caspase cascade would lead to abnormal expression of some key regulatory factors that may lead to cancer. The experimental evidence has indicated the intricate relationships between apoptosis and cancer.[7,8]

## Autophagy and cancer

Autophagy is catabolic mechanism highly regulated by some autophagy-related genes (ATGs) with many links to cellular activities that occur in malignant cells. It is a crucial mechanism that responds to either extra- or intracellular stress and can result in cell survival under certain circum-stances. However, over-activation of autophagy may result in autophagic cell death.[9] When examining relationships between autophagy and cancer, it is helpful to determine whether autophagy protects cell survival or contributes to cell death. Autophagy is well known to be crucial for cell survival and degradation of intracellular macromolecules that provide energy required for minimal cell functioning when nutrients are scarce.[10] Autophagic activation can play a protective role in early stages of cancer progression.[11] In contrast, however, autophagy can perform as a tumor suppressor by activating pro-autophagic genes and blocking anti-autophagic genes in oncogenesis. However, autophagy can also play a pro-tumor role in carcinogenesis through regulating a number of pathways involving Beclin-1, Bcl-2, Class III and I PI3K, Mammalian Target of Rapamycin (a protein)(mTOR) C1/C2, and p53.[11]

## Necrosis and cancer

Necrosis is an uncontrolled process of cell death. With the discovery of key mediators of necrotic death such as receptor-interacting protein (RIP) kinases and poly (ADP-ribose) polymerase-1 (PARP1), the activity of necrosis can be modulated. RIP kinases, PARP1, NADPH oxidases, and calpains have been identified as potential signaling components of programmed necrosis.[12,13] When cells undergo necrosis, integrity of the cell membrane is disrupted so that intracellular materials are released into the extracellular milieu, leading to inflammatory responses by immune cells, and local inflammation that may promote tumor growth.[14]

## Cross-talk among signaling pathways in apoptosis, autophagy, and necrosis

Apoptosis, autophagy, and necrosis bear distinct characteristics and physiological processes. However, there still exist intricate mechanistic actions between them. Under some circumstances, apoptosis and autophagy can exert synergetic effects, whereas in other situations, autophagy can be triggered only when apoptosis is suppressed.[4,15] Autophagy may act either as a guardian or as an executioner, relying on stage of carcinogenesis, the surrounding cellular environment, or therapeutic interventions.[16]

Necrosis is caspase-independent cell death, always triggered as a backup mechanism for apoptosis when caspases are inactivated.[17] However, the death mode can be switched due to conversion from mitochondrial inner membrane permeability to mitochondrial outer membrane permeability (MOMP) by specific stimulants.[18] Under certain conditions, apoptosis and necrosis are induced simultaneously and deficiency of both apoptosis and necrosis can be found in some cancer cells.[19]

## Signaling pathways in cancer

The DR family, which includes tumor necrosis factor receptor TNF-R1, Fas, DR3, TRAIL-R1/2(DR4/5), and DR6, can initiate the extrinsic pathway leading to apoptosis.[20-23] Members of the DR mainly rely on the in the cytoplasm, which when bound to their appropriate ligands recruit FADD. When pro-caspase-8 becomes hydrolyzed into active caspase-8, the recruited adaptor protein containing death effector domain (DED), can interact with DED of pro-caspases-8–10, thus aggregating as a DISC.[21] When stimuli occur as Fas combines with Fas-L, death complex recruiting FADD, and pro-caspase-8, formation of the DISC is initiated to activate caspase-8.[22,23]

## Bcl-2 family, regulators of apoptosis

The Bcl-2 family is overexpressed in many types of cancer cell.[24] Reduction of Bcl-2 expression may promote apoptotic responses to anticancer drugs. On the contrary, increased expression of Bcl-2 leads to resistance to chemotherapeutic drugs and radiation therapy. The whole Bcl-2 family is composed of a number of pro-apoptotic members such as Bax, Bak, Bad, Bcl-XS, Bid, Bik, Bim, and Hrk, plus anti-apoptotic members such as Bcl-2, Bcl-XL, Bcl-W, Bfl-1, and Mcl-1.[25] Pro-apoptotic proteins are able to undergo post-translational modifications that can lead to their activation and translocation to mitochondria, from which apoptosis can be initiated.[26] All BH3-only molecules require multidomain BH3 proteins including Bax and Bak to apply their intrinsic pro-apoptotic activities. These lead to release of cytochrome $c$ and activator of caspases; the outer mitochondrial membrane becomes permeable in response to apoptotic stimuli, while cytochrome $c$ can interact with Apaf-1 once released into the cytosol, leading to activation of caspase-9.[27] Activated caspase-9 activates caspase-3, and the downstream caspase cascade leading to apoptosis.

## Modulation of apoptosis

Caspase-9 is one of the most representative initiators of mitochondrial apoptosis. Apoptotic factors that induce DNA damage or inhibit DNA repair, pro-apoptotic BH3-only proteins Bim, Bid, and Bad can be activated, and promote oligomerization of p53 effector Bax/Bak, permeabilization of the mitochondrial outer membrane.[28,29] However, the expression of Bcl-2 family members Bcl-2, Bcl-XL, and Mcl-1 may be modulated to counteract this effect.[30] It has been reported that caspase-2, containing a caspase recruitment domain (CARD) and multi-protein complex, may mediate mitochondrial permeabilization by cleaving and activating Bid, when DNA damage has induced apoptosis.[31] In the cytoplasm, cytochrome $c$ binding to Apaf-1 in the presence of dATP or ATP promotes self-oligomerization of Apaf-1.[32] It is important to observe that both Apaf-1 and caspase-9 contain the protein interaction motif CARD, while Apaf-1 strongly binds caspase-9 through CARD–CARD interactions, leading to formation of a cytoplasmic feature called the apoptosome, then dimerization-induced activation of caspase-9.[33] WD40 repeat (WDR) domains of Apaf-1 recruit downstream executioners caspase-3 and caspase-7 as soon as the core complex is formed and caspase-9 is activated.[34] Downstream executioners cleave the targeted key regulatory molecule to bring about apoptotic cell death.[35]

## NF-jB

NF-jB is a class of protein with various transcriptional regulatory functions involved in apoptosis and tumorigenesis, and IKKbeta subunit of IkappaB kinase (IKK)/NF-jB in apoptosis were reported.[8,36] NF-jB activation is initiated by signal-induced degradation of IjB protein, which bind NF-jB acting as its inhibitor, resulting in its inactivation and to avoid apoptosis through subsequent transcriptional regulation. Inactivation of NF-jB pathways can promote apoptosis.[37]

## p53

The nuclear transcription factor p53 regulates apoptotic signals in the intrinsic pathway of apoptosis.[38] p53 is an important proapoptotic factor and tumor inhibitor. Anti-tumor agents drugs can be developed to modulate apoptosis by targeting p53-related signaling pathways. p53 promotes apoptotic cell death through DR-5 and Bax.[39]

## MicroRNAs in apoptosis

MicroRNAs (miRNAs) play pivotal roles in regulation of around 30% of gene expressions. Some tumor suppressors, such as the miR-15a-miR-16-1, miR-29, and let-7 family, can modulate core apoptotic pathways.[40] It has been reported that miR15-a and miR-16-1 trigger Bcl-2 to induce apoptosis, while Bcl-2 inhibits mitochondrial-mediated apoptosis through binding of Bax and Bak at the post-transcriptional level. Bcl-2 could regulate intrinsic apoptotic induction.

The let-7 family can initiate expression of proapoptotic protein Bim a caspase cascade leading to apoptosis. The MiR-34 family is a tumor suppressor, which activates the p53 expression to induce apoptosis.[41] Some miRNAs play their regulatory role as oncogenes, including miRNA-21, the miRNA-17-92 cluster, miRNA-221, -222, and miRNA-272, -273, to increase the rate of cancer cell proliferation.[42] Anti-apoptotic factor miRNA-21 has been found to upregulate miRNA in many types of cancer through the PCD 4 gene (PDCD4), phosphatase and tensin homologue (PTEN), and tropomyosin 1 (TPM1).[43] Regulation of PTEN by miR-21 has been observed to increase expression of Matrix metalloproteinases (MMPs) MMP-9 and MMP-2, in normal hepatocytes. In addition, PTEN has been known to be a therapeutic target of many miRNAs, including the miR-17-92 cluster, miR-214.[40] MiRNA-21 can also target TPM1, a member of the TPM protein family, which functions as a serpin peptidase inhibitor. In breast cancer, inhibition of miR-21 causes increase in TPM1 protein expression, involved in the 3-UTR of TPM1. A previous study suggested the let-7 family possibly co-operated with miR-21, functioning in cancer progression.[43]

# Autophagic pathways in cancer

## ULK1/2 and Atg13

In mammals, two homologues of Atg1 include ULK1 and ULK2. Atg13 and scaffold protein FIP200 (an orthologue of yeast Atg17) together are able to form a complex, while FIP200 can localize ULK to pre-autophagosomal structures for recruitment of other Atg proteins.[44] Atg13 binds to ULK and thus inhibiting autophagy.[45]

## PI3KCI-Akt-mTORC1

The PI3KCI-AKT-mTORC1 signaling pathway is believed to be associated with a series of cell processes and can be deregulated by various genetic and epigenetic mechanisms in a wide range of cancer cells.[46] Thus, the PI3KCI-Akt-mTOR pathway can be modulated. Akt is a protein serine/threonine kinase is known to induce development of cancers.[47] Signaling pathways that promote mTORC1 activity are induced by oncoproteins or loss of tumor suppressors, and thus mTORC1-inhibited autophagy is often observed in malignant cells. The results reported that PI3KCI inhibited autophagy by activation of the Akt pathway.[48] mTORC1 is believed to be activated in part by Akt through tuberous sclerosis complex proteins, TSC1 and TSC2, as the TSC1/TSC2 complex is a critical negative regulator of mTORC1.[49].

# Regulation of apoptosis through caspase activation

The regulation of apoptosis through caspases occurs by two distinct molecular signaling pathways, namely extrinsic and intrinsic pathways. The activation of caspases results from the formation of a multiprotein complex, termed the apoptosome, consisting of CED-4/Apaf-1, procaspase-9, and cytochrome *c* (in mammals only), which is required for the initial activation of procaspase-9, with the activation of other caspases occurring subsequent to caspase-9 activation.[50] Caspases that are activated downstream of caspase-9 participate in the degradation of the cellular components, such as caspase-3, an effector caspases. The disturbance of balance between pro-apoptotic and anti-apoptotic signaling events can induce apoptosis, which may be triggered by environmental (extracellular) factors, such as Fas ligand (FasL/CD95L), tumor necrosis factor a (TNFa), transforming growth factor b (TGFb), and cytokines. Most growth factors and cytokines promote cell growth and differentiation through anti-apoptotic signaling on their target cells. Mutations of growth factors can be mediated by targeted overexpression of anti-apoptotic factor Bcl-2.

In mammals, the extrinsic pathway mediates apoptosis in response to the activation of cell surface DRs, such as Fas/CD95 and TNFa receptor. DRs can induce apoptosis through the activation of caspases or through the activation of the intrinsic/mitochondrial pathway. Activated DRs bind to the adaptor molecule FADD via the DD and FADD recruits the initiator procaspase-8 and procaspase-10 into a complex, the DISC, through the DED, which is present both in FADD and in the procaspase. The sequential activation of caspase cascade leads to apoptosis.

# Role of the c-Myc

Role of the c-Myc oncogene is in the control of apoptosis. Additional factors have been shown to regulate apoptosis, including the proto-oncogene c-Myc, which has a central role in the regulation of growth control, cell differentiation, and apoptosis. It is among the genes that most frequently contribute to the development of human tumors. c-Myc is a transcription factor that recognizes the CA[C/T]GTG element (E box) and also has the ability to repress transcription through a pyrimidine-rich cis element termed the initiator (Inr). The target genes of c-Myc are involved in cell cycle regulation, metabolism, protein synthesis, and cell adhesion.

Overexpression of c-Myc has been found to promote apoptosis.[51–52] Inhibition of c-Myc resulted in dramatic apoptosis, whereas overexpression of c-Myc protected B cells from apoptosis. However, it appears that multiple pathways are regulated by Myc including one requiring the p53 tumor suppressor, where Myc-induced apoptosis is preceded by stabilization of p53. Apoptosis depends on the balance between proapoptotic and anti-apoptotic signaling components within cells. The understanding of these signaling pathways and molecular targets opens opportunities that may lead to specific cancer therapies and diseases caused by deregulation of the normal cell death processes.

# Active phytochemical compounds with sulfhydryl (R–SH) group

Most users of herbal medicine and healthcare products that contain herbal ingredients perceive that herbs are efficacious and can be more effective than conventional medicines. More importantly, it seldom induces significant cytotoxicity.

This perception may be a major contributing factor influencing the increasing popularity of herbs. Although herbs are often promoted as natural and therefore harmless, they contain phytochemical compounds that can be metabolized to produce toxic metabolites; thus, some of the herbal medicines may display adverse effects if not use under the supervision of Chinese medicine practitioners. Some of the chemical active ingredients cause cytotoxicity yet they exert beneficial effects on the body. The common active phytochemicals are shown in Table 5.1. Previous study indicated that herbal supplements are associated with adverse events that include all levels of organ toxicity.[53] However, dosage and purity of active compounds in herbal supplements are crucial to ameliorate potential toxicity. Moreover, another report showed that 21% of older adults took more than one herbal product or dietary supplement, and potential for adverse drug reactions is apparent in 19% of respondents.[54] Therefore, the current popularity of herbal products renders necessarily the evaluation of their biochemical activity and safety of the products. In addition, within the fields of pharmacology and biochemistry, a drug or a substrate of drug-metabolizing enzymes should be a small size natural product or regulator that is able to enter cells easily because it has a low molecular weight. Once inside the cells, it can affect other cellular molecules, such as proteins, DNAase,

**Table 5.1**  Common active phytochemical compounds with sulfhydryl (R–SH) group.

| Compound | Action | Reference |
|---|---|---|
| Sulforaphane | • Inhibits breast cancer stem cells (CSCs) and down-regulates Wnt/β-catenin self-renewal pathway<br>• →Chemoprevention of breast CSCs | Nabekura *et al.*[55], Li *et al.*[56] |
| 6-Methylsulfinyl hexyl isothiocyanate | • Anti-inflammatory, anti-microbial, antiplatelet, and anticancer effects<br>• Strongly suppresses cyclooxygenase-2 (COX-2), inducible nitric oxide synthase (iNOS), and cytokines, which are important factors that mediate inflammatory processes<br>• Anticancer activity against the growth and CSC phenotypes of human pancreatic cancer cells | Nabekura *et al.*[55], Uto *et al.*[57], Chen *et al.*[58] |
| Diallyl sulfide/diallyl trisulfide | • Anticancer effect | Nabekura *et al.*[55], Seki *et al.*[59] |
| S-allylmercaptocysteine | • Antimetastatic agent for the treatment of androgen-independent prostate cancer<br>• Inhibits the proliferation of colorectal cancer cells | Aggarwal and Shishodia[60], Howard *et al.*[61], Liang *et al.*[62] |

| Compound | Action | Reference |
|---|---|---|
| Ajoene | Anti-thrombosis, anti-microbial, and cholesterol-lowering activities | Aggarwal and Shishodia[60], Hassan[63] |
| Allicin | Inhibit the proliferation and induce apoptosis of several human non-leukemia malignant cells including breast, bladder, colorectal, hepatic, prostate cancer, lymphoma, and skin tumor cell lines | Hassan[63] |

and polymerase, and may modulate signaling processes that are associated with cancer growth. Some common small size molecules are listed in Appendix II. Many targeted therapies are small molecule drugs or small molecule inhibitors. Small size natural products are better drug candidates.

# References

1. Ouyang, L., Shi, Z., Zhao, S., *et al.* (2012). Programmed cell death pathways in cancer: a review of apoptosis, autophagy and programmed necrosis. *Nat Med.* 45(6): 487–498.
2. Kaleigh, F., and Kurokawa, M.K. (2013). Evading apoptosis in cancer. Trends Cell Biol. 23(12): 620–633.
3. Ouyang, L., Shi, Z., Zhao, S., et al. (2012). Programmed cell death pathways in cancer: a review of apoptosis, autophagy and programmed necrosis. *Cell Prolif.* 45: 487–498. doi: 10.1111/j.1365-2184.2012.00845.x
4. Amelio, I., Melino, G., and Knight, R.A. (2011). Cell death pathology: cross-talk with autophagy and its clinical implications. *Biochem Biophys Res Commun.* 414: 277–281.
5. Eum, K.H., and Lee, M. (2011). Crosstalk between autophagy and apoptosis in the regulation of paclitaxel-induced cell death in v-Ha-ras-transformed fibroblasts. *Mol Cell Biochem.* 348: 61–68.
6. Nishida, K., Yamaguchi, O., and Otsu, K. (2008). Crosstalk between autophagy and apoptosis in heart disease. *Circ Res.* 103: 343–351.
7. Kerr, J.F.R., Wyllie, A.H., and Currie, A.R. (1982). Apoptosis: a basic biological phenomenon with wide-ranging implications in tissue kinetics. *Br J Cancer.* 26: 239–257.
8. Ghobrial, I.M., Witzig, T.E., and Adjei, A.A. (2005). Targeting apoptosis pathways in cancer therapy. *Cancer J Clin.* 55: 178–194.
9. Wang, S.Y., Yu, Q.J., Zhang, R.D., and Liu, B. (2011). Core signaling pathways of survival/death in autophagy-related cancer networks. *Int J Biochem Cell Biol.* 43: 1263–1266.

10. White, E. (2012). Deconvoluting the context-dependent role for autophagy in cancer. *Nat Rev Cancer.* 12: 401–410.

11. Kundu, M., and Thompson, C.B. (2008). Autophagy: basic principles and relevance to disease. *Annu Rev Pathol.* 3: 427–455.

12. Galluzzi, L., and Kroemer, G. (2008). Necroptosis: a specialized pathway of programmed necrosis. *Cell.* 135: 1161–1163.

13. Golstein, P., and Kroemer, G. (2007). Cell death by necrosis: towards a molecular definition. *Trends Biochem Sci.* 32: 37–43.

14. Zong, W.X., Ditsworth, D., Bauer, D.E., Wang, Z.Q., and Thompson, C.B. (2004). Alkylating DNA damage stimulates a regulated form of necrotic cell death. *Genes Dev.* 18: 1272–1282.

15. Gonzalez-Polo, R.A., Boya, P., Pauleau, A.L., Jalil, A., Larochette, N., and Souquere, S. (2005). The apoptosis/autophagy paradox: autophagic vacuolization before apoptotic death. *J Cell Sci.* 118: 3091–3102.

16. Michels, J., Kepp, O., Senovilla, L., *et al.* (2013). Functions of BCL-X L at the interface between cell death and metabolism. *Int J Cell Biol.* 2013: 705294. doi: 10.1155/2013/705294

17. Degterev, A., Huang, Z., Boyce, M., Li, Y., Jagtap, P., and Mizushima, N. (2005). Chemical inhibitor of nonapoptotic cell death with therapeutic potential for ischemic brain injury. *Nat Chem Biol.* 1: 112–119.

18. Han, W., Xie, J., Li, L., Liu, Z., and Hu, X. (2009). Necrostatin-1 reverts shikonin-induced necroptosis to apoptosis. *Apoptosis.* 14: 674–686.

19. Liu, P., Xu, B., Shen, W., Zhu, H., Wu, W., and Fu, Y. (2012). Dysregulation of TNF-α-induced necroptotic signaling in chronic lymphocytic: suppression of CYLD gene by LEF1. *Leukemia.* 26: 1293–1300.

20. Sayers, T.J. (2011). Targeting the extrinsic apoptosis signaling pathway for cancer therapy. *Cancer Immunol Immunother.* 60: 1173–1180.

21. Mannick, J.B., Hausladen, A., Liu, L., Hess, D.T., Zeng, M., and Miao, Q.X. (1999). Fas-induced caspase denitrosylation. *Science.* 284: 651–654.

22. Sun, S.Y. (2011). Understanding the role of the death receptor 5/FADD/caspase-8 death signaling in cancer metastasis. *Mol Cell Pharmacol.* 3: 31–34.

23. Bell, B.D., Leverrier, S., Weist, B.M., Newton, R.H., Arechiga, A.F., and Luhrs, K.A. (2008). FADD and caspase-8 control the outcome of autophagic signaling in proliferating T cells. *Proc Natl Acad Sci USA.* 105: 16677–16682.

24. Llambi, F., and Green, D.R. (2011). Apoptosis and oncogenesis: give and take in the BCL-2 family. *Curr Opin Genet Dev.* 21: 12–20.

25. Engel, T., and Henshall, D.C. (2009). Apoptosis, Bcl-2 family proteins and caspases: the ABCs of seizure-damage and epileptogenesis? *Int J Physiol Pathophysiol Pharmacol.* 1: 97–115.

26. Shamas-Din, A., Brahmbhatt, H., Leber, B., and Andrews, D.W. (2011). BH3-only proteins: orchestrators of apoptosis. *Biochim Biophys Acta.* 1813: 508–520.

27. Wen, X., Lin, Z.Q., Liu, B., and Wei, Y.Q. (2012). Caspase-mediated programmed cell death pathways as potential therapeutic targets in cancer. *Cell Prolif.* 45: 217–224.

28. Zou, H., Henzel, W.J., Liu, X., Lutschg, A., and Wang, X. (1997). Apaf-1, a human protein homologous to C. elegans CED-4, participates in cytochrome c-dependent activation of caspase-3. *Cell.* 90: 405–413.

29. Li, P., Nijhawan, D., Budihardjo, I., Srinivasula, S.M., Ahmad, M., and Alnemri, E.S. (1997). Cytochrome c and dATP-dependent formation of Apaf-1/caspase-9 complex initiates an apoptotic protease cascade. *Cell.* 91: 479–489.
30. Kelly, P.N., and Strasser, A. (2011). The role of Bcl-2 and its pro-survival relatives in tumourigenesis and cancer therapy. *Cell Death Differ.* 18: 1414–1424.
31. Ghavami, S., Hashemi, M., Ande, S.R., Yeganeh, B., Xiao, W., and Eshraghi, M. (2009). Caspase genes apoptosis and cancer: mutations within caspase genes. *Am J Med Genet.* 46: 497–510.
32. Scaffidi, C., Fulda, S., Srinivasan, A., Friesen, C., Li, F., and Tomaselli, K.J. (1998). Two CD95 (APO-1/Fas) signaling pathways. *EMBO J.* 17: 1675–1687.
33. Kurokawa, M., and Kornbluth, S. (2009). Caspases and kinases in a death grip. *Cell.* 138: 838–854.
34. Giansanti, V., Torriglia, A., and Scovassi, A.I. (2011). Conversation between apoptosis and autophagy: "Is it your turn or mine?" *Apoptosis.* 16: 321–333.
35. Allan, L.A., and Clarke, P.R. (2009). Apoptosis and autophagy: regulation of caspase-9 by phosphorylation. *FEBS J.* 276: 6063–6073.
36. Karin, M., and Greten, F.R. (2005). NF-kappaB: linking inflammation and immunity to cancer development and progression. *Nat Rev Immunol.* 5: 749–759.
37. Karin, M., Yamamoto, Y., and Wang, Q.M. (2004). The IKK NF-jB system: a treasure trove for drug development. *Nat Rev Drug Discov.* 3: 17–26.
38. Kastan, M.B., Onyekwere, O., Sidransky, D., Vogelstein, B., and Craig, R.W. (1991). Participation of p53 protein in the cellular response to DNA damage. *Cancer Res.* 51: 6304–6311.
39. Yu, J., Wang, Z., Kinzler, K.W., Vogelstein, B., and Zhang, L. (2003). PUMA mediates the apoptotic response to p53 in colorectal cancer cells. *Proc Natl Acad Sci USA.* 100: 1931–1936.
40. Lima, R.T., Busacca, S., Almeida, G.M., Gaudino, G., Fennell, D.A., and Vasconcelos, M.H. (2011). MicroRNA regulation of core apoptosis pathways in cancer. *Eur J Cancer.* 47: 163–174.
41. Miller, T.E., Ghoshal, K., Ramaswamy, B., Roy, S., Datta, J., and Shapiro, C.L. (2008). MicroRNA-221/222 confers tamoxifen resistance in breast cancer by targeting p27Kip1. *J Biol Chem.* 283: 29897–29903.
42. Linnstaedt, S.D., Gottwein, E., Skalsky, R.L., Luftig, M.A., and Cullen, B.R. (2010). Virally induced cellular microRNA miR-155 plays a key role in B-cell immortalization by Epstein-Barr virus. *J Virol.* 84: 11670–11678.
43. Wang, Y., and Lee, C.G. (2009). MicroRNA and cancer — focus on apoptosis. *J Cell Mol Med.* 13: 12–23.
44. Hara, T., Takamura, A., Kishi, C., Iemura, S., Natsume, T., and Guan, J.L. (2008). FIP200, a uLK-interacting protein, is required for autophagosome formation in mammalian cells. *J Cell Biol.* 181: 497–510.
45. Hosokawa, N., Hara, T., Kaizuka, T., Kishi, C., Takamura, A., and Miura, Y. (2009). Nutrient-dependent mTORC1 association with the uLK1-Atg13-FIP200 complex required for autophagy. *Mol Biol Cell.* 7: 1981–1991.
46. Weinstein, I.B., and Joe, A.K. (2006). Mechanisms of disease: oncogene addiction — a rationale for molecular targeting in cancer therapy. *Nat Clin Pract Oncol.* 3: 448–457.

47. Loewith, R., Jacinto, E., Wullschleger, S., Lorberg, A., Crespo, J.L., and Bonenfant, D. (2002). Two TOR complexes, only one of which is rapamycin sensitive, have distinct roles in cell growth control. *Mol Cell.* 10: 457–468.

48. Akca, H., Demiray, A., Aslan, M., Acikbas, I., and Tokgun, O. (2012). Tumour suppressor PTEN enhanced enzyme activity of GPx, SOD and catalase by suppression of PI3K/AKT pathway in non-small cell lung cancer cell lines. *J Enzyme Inhib Med Chem.* 28(3): 539–544. doi: 10.3109/14756366.2011.654114

49. Brugarolas, J., Lei, K., Hurley, R.L., Manning, B.D., Reiling, J.H., and Hafen, E. (2004). Regulation of mTOR function in response to hypoxia by REDD1 and the TSC1/TSC2 tumor suppressor complex. *Genes Dev.* 18: 2893–2904.

50. Shi, Y. (2006). Mechanical aspects of apoptosome assembly. *Curr Opin Cell Biol.* 18: 677–684.

51. Hoffman, B., and Liebermann, D.A. (2008). Apoptotic signaling by c-MYC. *Oncogene.* 27: 6462–6472.

52. Borrelli, F., Capasso, R., and Angelo, A. (2007). IzzoGarlic (Allium sativum L.): adverse effects and drug. *Mol Nutr Food Res.* 51: 1386–1397.

53. Palmer, M.E., Haller, C., McKinney, P.E., and Klein-Schwartz, W. (2003). Adverse events associated with dietary supplements: an observational study. *Lancet.* 361: 101–106.

54. Marinac, J.S., Buchinger, C.L., Godfrey, L.A., and Wooten, J.M. (2007). Herbal products and dietary supplements: a survey of use, attitudes, and knowledge among older adults. *J Am Osteopath Assoc.* 107: 13–20.

55. Nabekura, T., Kamiyama, S., and Kitagawa, S. (2005). Effects of dietary chemopreventive phytochemicals on P-glycoprotein function. *Biochem Biophys Res Commun.* 327(3): 866–870.

56. Li, Y., Zhang, T., Korkaya, H., *et al.* (2010). Sulforaphane, a dietary component of broccoli/broccoli sprouts, inhibits breast cancer stem cells. *Clin Cancer Res.* 16(9): 2580–2590.

57. Uto, T., Hou, D.X., Morinaga, O., and Shoyama, Y. (2010). Molecular mechanisms underlying anti-inflammatory actions of 6-(Methylsulfinyl)hexyl isothiocyanate derived from Wasabi (*Wasabia japonica*). *Adv Pharmacol Sci.* 2010: 614046.

58. Chen, Y.J., Huang, Y.C., Tsai, T.H., and Liao, H.F. (2014). Effect of Wasabi component 6-(Methylsulfinyl)hexyl isothiocyanate and derivatives on human pancreatic cancer cells. *Evid Based Complement Altern Med.* 2014: 494739.

59. Seki, T., Hosono, T., Hosono-Fukao, T., *et al.* (2008). Anticancer effects of diallyl trisulfide derived from garlic. *Asia Pac J Clin Nutr.* 17(Suppl 1): 249–252.

60. Aggarwal, B.B., and Shishodia, S. (2004). Suppression of the nuclear factor-kappa B activation pathway by spice-derived phytochemicals — reasoning for seasoning. *Ann N Y Acad Sci.* 1030: 434–441.

61. Howard, E.W., Ling, M.T., Chua, C.W., Cheung, H.W., Wang, X., and Wong, Y.C. (2007). Garlic-derived S-allylmercaptocysteine is a novel in vivo antimetastatic agent for androgen-independent prostate cancer. *Clin Cancer Res.* 13(6): 1847–1856.

62. Liang, D., Qin, Y., Zhao, W., *et al.* (2011). S-allylmercaptocysteine effectively inhibits the proliferation of colorectal cancer cells under in vitro and in vivo conditions. *Cancer Lett.* 310(1): 69–76.

63. Hassan, H.T. (2004). Ajoene (natural garlic compound): a new anti-leukaemia agent for AML therapy. *Leuk Res.* 28(7): 667–671.

# INTEGRATION AND CONTROL OF THE HUMAN BODY DURING TREATMENT

Although traditional Chinese medicine (TCM) has been commonly used by Chinese practitioners to treat ailments including cancer, the effectiveness of combining TCM with Western medicine in managing cancer has not been evaluated scientifically and systematically. A previous study showed clinical effectiveness of combining TCM and Western medicine in the treatment of irritable bowel syndrome (IBS). Compared with the Western medicine treatment alone, the result showed TCM combined with Western interventions significantly improved IBS global symptoms (risk ratio (RR), 1.21; 95% Interstitial cystitis pain (CI): 1.18–1.24).[1] Both Chinese proprietary herbal medicine plus conventional treatment and herbal preparations plus conventional treatment showed similar and statistically significant effects on IBS compared with western treatment alone. These results demonstrated that treating IBS with integrated traditional Chinese and Western medicines showed better effectiveness than conventional Western medicine alone. TCM, particularly Chinese proprietary medicine with the benefits of low-cost and good palatability, would be an attractive option to be used in conjunction with conventional Western medicine to manage other diseases and cancer.[1]

## Persistent pain

Frozen shoulder is a common disorder, characterized by spontaneous onset of pain in the shoulder and accompanied by limitation of glenohumeral movement. Treatments for frozen shoulder include physical therapy, corticosteroid injection, and arthroscopic capsular release. Several patients suffer from some degree of pain and range-of-motion limitation for up to 10 years even when these treatments are applied. Kampo and Nijutsuto, a Japanese herbal medicine based on traditional Chinese herbal medicine, have been used for the treatment of pain in Japan. Thirteen patients suffering from long-term frozen shoulder refractory to Western medical treatment were administered Nijutsuto. It was reported that almost all patients experienced pain relief after Nijutsuto administration.[2]

## TCM in the era of evidence-based medicine

Evidence-based medicine (EBM), by integrating Chinese medicine (CM) practitioners' expertise with clinical evidence from systematic research, has established platform for the standard of modern medical practice for efficacy and safety of TCM.[3] TCM has evolved as a system of medical practice from ancient China more than 2000 years ago based on empirical knowledge and theories, which are yet to be mapped by scientific equivalents. Despite the expanding TCM usage and the recognition of its therapeutic benefits worldwide, the lack of scientific and systemic evidence from the EBM perspective remains hardly acceptable by the Western medicine community and its integration into mainstream healthcare. For TCM to become an integral component of the healthcare products, it is essential for TCM to demonstrate with scientific evidence. It is worth exploring evidences available on its efficacy and safety and highlight challenges faced in applying EBM to TCM.

## Integrating TCM healthcare into diabetes care

The TCM formula Liu-Wei-Di-Huang-Wan, which consists of six types of herbs, namely *Rehmannia glutinosa* (Gaertn.) DC., root, dried; *Cornus officinalis* Siebold & Zucc., fructus, dried; *Dioscorea oppositifolia* L., root, dried; *Alisma plantago-aquatica* subsp. orientale (Sam.) Sam., tuber, dried; Paeonia × suffruticosa Andrews, bark, dried; Poriacocos (Fr.) Wolf., sclerotium, dried, is one of the most frequently prescribed herbal medicine used to treat type 2 diabetes patients.[4] The integration of TCM into diabetes care showed it reduces the risk of developing kidney failure. The Taiwan's National Health Insurance Research Database (NHIRD) provided information of healthcare services for each patient in 2007.[4] Case and control subjects were selected from the NHIRD. Two multivariable logistic regression models were employed to explore two types of exposure assessments including prescription of TCMs (model 1) and prescription of different estimated dosages of Liu-Wei-Di-Huang-Wan (model 2). Using logistic regression model 1, the results showed that TCMs were associated with a decreased risk of kidney failure by multivariable analysis (odds ratio (OR) = 0.69, 95% CI: 0.61–0.77). There was no difference between non-Liu-Wei-Di-Huang-Wan TCM users and Liu-Wei-Di-Huang-Wan TCM users in terms of the risk of developing kidney failure. Furthermore, there was also no linear dose–response trend when we used exposure to prescribed Liu-Wei-Di-Huang-Wan as a continuous variable (for non-Liu-Wei-Di-Huang-Wan TCM users, OR = 0.68, 95% CI: 0.60–0.77; for TCM users consuming 1–30 g of Liu-Wei-Di-Huang-Wan, OR = 0.69, 95% CI: 0.54–0.87; and for >30 g of Liu-Wei-Di-Huang-Wan, OR = 0.84, 95% CI: 0.49–1.44). Integrating TCM healthcare into patient care was found to be useful and fruitful. The study enables us to explore potential interactions and adverse effects with the formulations on treatment strategy that may be beneficial to patients.

## TCM formulations in cancer therapy

CM has been used to prevent and treat diseases including cancer for several thousand years. However, the lack of scientific evidences has hampered the practice of the integrated approach to cancer therapy. In the recent four decades, a number of CM herbs have aroused great interest in developing anticancer compounds from medicinal herbs. Some of these active compounds exhibit a variety of biological responses and inhibitory effects on cancer including angiogenesis inhibitors.[5] The results showed both the experimental and clinical assessments obtained in the field of clinical oncology. The study also presents the promise of integration of CM and drugs in basic research and clinical practice when CM was used as adjuvant and maintenance therapy.

## Dilemma with combination therapy

A previous study reported different perspectives of the TCM practitioners and Western medicine and explored the possible ways of integration of TCM and Western medicine in treatment of diseases.[6] It was reported that the integrated medicine was applied to evaluate the safety and efficacy of TCM I combination with Western medicine. Qualitative design was based on focus group interviews of TCM practitioners in Hong Kong, and participants were recruited from a Western medicine training course for TCM practitioners. Two focus groups comprising 13 TCM practitioners were held before the course and two others with 10 TCM practitioners after the course. The TCM practitioners were adapted to act in a supportive role to Western doctors. They highlighted the prejudice from the Western doctors on their diagnostic approach. The TCM practitioners felt that they were actually more open minded than the Western doctors, who often discouraged the patients to see them. They considered Western medicine as a complicated issue due to the different concepts and forms of integration. Western medicine might overweigh the TCM. Yet TCM remains hard to be integrated with Western medicine over the centuries. The TCM practitioners are more flexible to the healthcare system for patients. Despite the hurdles for integration with Western medicine, the TCM practitioners tend to support the trend of integration.

## Co-administration of Western drugs and herbal medicines

Use of complementary and alternative medicine (CAM) is increasing worldwide. Herb–drug interactions can occur when it is not administered properly due probably of interactions of drug metabolites and active compounds of herbal medicine, which may influence the therapeutic benefits of co-administered allopathic medicines.[7] Although valuable information on herb–drug interactions is obtained by *in vitro* and *in vivo* studies, the mechanism of interaction remains sketchy.[7] The results, however, suggested the potential toxicity of the interactions. Furthermore, the results also suggested herb–drug interactions problems with co-administration of drugs and TCM especially with herbal formulations. More basic and clinical studies should be conducted to provide a better understanding of interactions between drugs and herbs. This would provide a platform for development of guidelines for co-administration of drugs and herbal medicine.

With the increasing use of TCM in combination of drugs for treatment of diseases and the unique advantages in healthcare in Europe, the United States, and many Asian countries, the effectiveness of the combination therapy becomes the focus of research in TCM. According to statistics, in the United States alone, there are currently more than 15 million people using herbal preparations in varying degrees, including Chinese herbal medicines, as either a therapy or an adjuvant therapy for various diseases at present, with the annual cost of approximately 30 billion USD.[8]

# Interactions between TCMs and Western therapeutics

TCM is an essential part of the healthcare system in several Asian countries and is considered a complementary or alternative medical system in most Western countries. An integration of the traditional Chinese and Western systems of medicine has begun in multiple medical centers internationally, and there is increasing evidence that several herbs and combinations of herbs used in TCM impart important pharmacological effects.[9] The number of databases and compilations of herbs, herbal formulations, phytochemical constituents, and molecular targets is increasing, primarily because of the widespread use of TCM in combination with Western drugs. The results suggested that evidence-based efficacy and safety of phytochemical constituents in herbs and TCM formulations are essential. Advancement in the knowledge of the molecular targets and metabolic pathways, as well as of the synergistic and inhibitory effects associated with important phytochemicals from herbs and herbal formulations, will lead to the development of rational approaches for the safe combination of healthcare systems from different cultures.

# Role of TCM in Western medicine

When the treatment methods for mind and body with combination of TCM and Western medicine are considered, a different concept could emerge that drastically changes the approach toward treatment of illness.[10] It is interesting to note that the combination of TCM and Western medicine in the early days in China preceded the Western model of integrated medicine by almost 50 years.[11] CM has played an important role in advancing integrated medicine. However, one of the major differences between the CM and the Western medicine lies on the scientific data to provide support of integrated medicine. The therapeutic integrated methods and their applications are not standardized. However, they are most frequently employed to treat chronic diseases, e.g., cancer, rheumatic disease, chronic inflammatory bowel disorder, chronic pain, and psychiatric problems including anxiety and depression. Nevertheless, the application of integrated medicine is limited by the availability of scientific data and clinical assessments of patients undergoing the combination therapy.

## Rationale for applying CM as chronotherapy against cancer

Current Western medical treatment relies on evidence-based medicine (EBM), and its effectiveness is quantitatively assessed based on treatment statistical methods. In contrast, cure or not is generally assessed by evaluating the patient's whole body functions. It is believed that TCM cannot be evaluated precisely according to Western principles, in which a constant amount of the same medicine is given to a group of patients to be evaluated.[10] When assessing cure using TCM, the balance of body functions and Yin-Yang is more important than the determination of medical effects. This means that quantitative evaluation of TCM treatment can be conducted qualitatively. A previous study was focused on the Yin-Yang balance to determine the medical effects and at the same time attempted to determine the treatment effects by applying the concept of regulation of Yin-Yang according to chronotherapeutic principles.[10] The study reported that advanced cancer patients generally lack both Yin and Yang. Chinese medical treatment therefore seeks to supplement both Yin and Yang. Yang (Qi) (cf. Glossary) tonic herbal treatment during the daytime, while the other group was administered Yin (Blood) (cf. Glossary) tonics during nighttime. A comparison of the results of treatment showed that the patients in the group receiving Yang (Qi) with tonic herbal replenishment during the daytime lived longer than patients receiving Yin (tonics) nourishment during the night. Moreover, the patients in the daytime Yang (Qi) replenishment group also fared significantly better than patients treated solely by Western methods.

## Integration of CM into supportive cancer care

An earlier study suggested that many traditional Chinese medical therapies were effective for the supportive care of cancer patients.[12] The results showed that integration of TCM with Western medicine did not provide evidence, which support further research into a developing model of integrative care. The holistic approach of TCM may be integrated into conventional Western medicine to supplement deficiencies in the current cancer therapy. The philosophy of TCM proposes novel hypotheses, which will support the development of a science-based holistic medicine.[12]

## A Strategy to uncover the anticancer mechanism of Chinese compound formula by integrating systems pharmacology and bioinformatics

Currently, cancer has become one of the major refractory diseases threatening human health. CAM has become a common alternative choice for patients due to the high cost of cancer therapy including surgery, radiotherapy, and chemotherapy. TCM has commonly used in preventing and treating cancer over the past few decades. Huanglian Jiedu Decoction (HJD), a classical Chinese compound formula, has been recognized to exert a beneficial effect on cancer patients with few adverse effects.[13] However, the mechanism of HJD remains unclear. An integrated methodology based on pharmacology and bioinformatics was used to explore the mechanistic actions of major active ingredients against cancer. The molecular targets were scrutinized using web-based Gene SeT Analysis Toolkit (WebGestalt), and 10 Kyoto Encyclopedia of Genes and Genomes (KEGG) pathways were identified by enrichment analysis. The results showed that the refined analysis of the KEGG pathways indicated that the anticancer effect of HJD displayed a functional correlation with the p53 signaling pathway; moreover, HJD had potential therapeutic effect on prostate cancer (PCa) and small cell lung cancer (SCLC).[13] Afterward, genetic alterations and survival analysis of key targets for cancer treatment were examined in both PCa and SCLC.[13] The results suggested that the integrated strategy provides a platform for future research on Chinese compound formula. The strategy contributes to reveal the anticancer effect and the mechanisms of action of Chinese compound formula.

## Integration of microRNA–mRNA profiles in cancer

A recent study showed that berberine is a bioactive alkaloid that can be isolated from several Chinese herbs, such as Huang lian (Rhizoma Coptidis). Rhizoma Coptidis was used in formations for treatment ailments including gastroenteritis and found that it could fight against tumors. The study was focused on integrating miRNA sequencing and RNA sequencing of cell line name (SGC-7901) gastric cancer cells treated by berberine to elucidate their underlying mechanisms.[14] The results showed that berberine inhibited the proliferation of SGC-7901 cells and induce G1 arrest in cell cycle phase and apoptosis. A total of 1,960 upregulated genes and 4,837 downregulated genes were identified in the RNA sequencing and 347 upregulated and 93 downregulated miRNAs in the miRNA sequencing. A total of 78 novel miRNAs were also found. Gene ontology and KEGG analysis showed that the genes were related to pathways in cancer and metabolism. Also, the miRNA–mRNA network of genes were grouped into cell cycle, apoptosis, inflammation, metabolism process, transforming growth factor (TGF-β) pathway, and Wnt signaling pathway. Integrated analysis of microRNA–mRNA profiles is a promising approach to validate gene expression patterns associated with malignancy and the mechanistic actions of anticancer agents. It has been reported that berberine is effective against a number of diseases including hyperlipidemia, diabetes, metabolic syndrome, and Alzheimer's disease, and a growing number of reports show that name of new drug (BBR is a substance that is being studied in the treatment of cancer) has anticancer effects.[15-18] However, the diversity of berberine targets has not been well understood yet. It has been reported that berberine regulated gene expression by targeting TATA boxes in transcriptional regulatory regions as well as the poly(A) tail at the mRNA terminus leading to apoptosis.[14] Recent researches have shown that BBR could also regulate the expression of miRNAs in several diseases.[17,18]

## Integration of phytochemicals and phytotherapy in cancer therapy

Concepts of individualized therapy in the 1970s and 1980s attempted to develop *in vitro* tests for individual drug responsiveness.[19] Individual medicine is to device specific cancer therapy strategies based on the health status of individuals and bioinformatics on drugs. However, tumor heterogeneity challenges chemotherapy due to genetic variations in cell populations, which may lead to refractory tumors. Natural products always served as vital resources for cancer therapy and are also sources for novel drug development. Targeted drugs are developed to interact with specific molecular targets and tumor-related proteins. Natural products from plants represent excellent resource for targeted therapies. Phytochemicals and herbal mixtures act on multiple targets and signaling pathways related to cancer. Drug resistance may be better understood by integrating phytochemicals and phytotherapy into Western medicine based on gene expression and network pharmacology. Different treatment modalities such as cytotoxic and targeted chemotherapy can be developed. Thereby, the use of big data analysis of TCM and phytotherapy represents an alternative approach to cancer therapy. The integration of phytochemicals and phytotherapy into cancer precision medicine offers a valuable platform for drug development and therapeutic antibodies.

## Resistance to anticancer drugs

Drug resistance was known in the early days of cancer chemotherapy more than half a century ago.[20,21] Drug resistance still hampers treatment of patients nowadays. Many of the common anticancer drugs come with drug toxicity and side effects. Thereby, the application of TCM in combination with Western drugs for cancer therapy has become a promising strategy to reduce severe side effects in cancer patients. As a consequence, an appropriate combination of phytochemicals from TCM and drug doses should be used.

Current chemotherapy protocols are effective. However, drug toxicity and the cellular response of each type of tumors vary and the treatment efficacy of individual patients cannot be reliably predicted yet the statistical probability of treatment response for larger groups of patients can be estimated from the results of clinical trials due to a substantial heterogeneity in cell population.[19] Drug resistance is a major obstacle in cancer therapy even though intensive cancer research is being performed. Although the molecular mechanism of drug resistance can be predicted, whether or not an individual tumor would respond in a similar manner to drug therapy remains sketchy.[22] Whereas sensitivity or resistance to targeted drugs can be compromised with an appropriate dosage, the outcome of treatment efficacy for the cytotoxic drugs is much more complicated, since their cellular targets frequently vary and these kinds of cytostatic drugs suggest broader modes of action against malignant and even normal proliferating cells.[19]

## The role of phytochemicals in drug development

Natural products always served as vital resources for cancer therapy. The therapeutic effects of plant-derived alkaloids were demonstrated with inhibition of the microtubule, the DNA topoisomerase I, and the podophyllotoxin-derived lignans, etoposide, and teniposide.[19] A previous report showed that a survey of the National Cancer Institute showed that 69% of anticancer drugs approved between the 1980s and 2002 were either natural products or natural products-derived agents.[23] Over 75% plant-derived drugs in clinical use nowadays are originated in traditional phytomedicine. Medicinal herbs belonged to the established repertoire to combat diseases. They are gaining relevance with increasing successes of synthetic pharmaceuticals in drug development during the 20th century.[24] Medicinal plants and other natural resources from marine or microbiological ecosystems become an excellent source of drug development. Secondary metabolites synthesized by plants serve as a defense against competitors, herbivores, and pathogens. These natural products and metabolites maintain crucial functions for survival and reproductive fitness of plants.[25] In addition to toxicity, secondary plant metabolites exert pharmacological features, which make them valuable for treatment of ailments in humans. The separation of these beneficial from harmful effects has become the main interest in research in toxicology and pharmacology of natural products.[26]

## Targeting tumor-related proteins with active natural products

The drawback with chemotherapy is that drugs cannot distinguish between normal and malignant cells. Any dividing cells can be attacked by the drugs. In order to enhance chemotherapy, drugs need to be more specific. Targeted drugs are designed to kill cancer cells by binding to the specific molecular target of cancer cells. Proteinomics and cytogenetic methods are employed for the drug development. Specific drug target is present only in tumor cells that bear amplified genes leading to protein overexpression. Also, chromosomal translocations may generate coding fusion genes for novel proteins that do not exist in healthy cells. Some of these aberrantly expressed genes trigger the development of cancer. Other genetic aberrations occur in the course of tumor progression.[27] Targeted drugs are specifically developed to mediate gene expression of proteins related to cancer. Instead of established therapy regimens for management of cancer patients with the same tumor type, targeted drugs can be developed based on the specific expression of aberrant targets in patients.

Two main categories of targeted drugs have been developed[19]:

(1) Monoclonal antibodies that can specifically interact with cell surface proteins. Examples are cetuximab and panitumumab against the epidermal growth factor receptor (EGFR), bevacizumab against vascular endothelial growth factor (VEGF), and rituximab against CD20.

(2) Small molecules that can be transported to the molecular targets in cancer cells, e.g., cancer-related kinases, imatinib mesylate is an example of targeted drug that inhibits the oncogenic breakpoint cluster region protein (BCR)/Abelson murine leukemia viral oncogene homolog 1 also known as (ABL) fusion protein. Other small molecules are erlotinib and gefitinib against EGFR, vemurafenib against proto-oncogene B-Raf (BRAF), and bortezomib against the proteasome.

Research in targeted therapy is undergoing rapid development. As more novel targets are being identified by tumor DNA sequencing and proteinomics, novel drugs can be developed. The economic impact of precision medicine in cancer therapy can be enormous in the years to come. Yet targeted drugs have considerable disadvantages:

(1) Alterations in the molecular target with point mutations, cell cycle arrest, related signaling pathways may cause ineffectiveness of targeted drug.[27]

(2) Targeted drugs also induced side effects in the body due to non-specific interactions. Side effects of targeted therapy are known to cause hepatotoxicity, dermatotoxicity, and hypertension.

Natural products may serve as lead compounds that can be chemically modified to produce derivatives with improved pharmacological properties.[28–31] The side effects of cytotoxic drugs and targeted therapy may be alleviated or abolished by natural products when used with cancer drugs. An earlier study demonstrated the potential of natural products for targeted therapy.[32,33] Signal transducer and activator of transcription 3 (STAT3) is an important molecule in signal transduction processes of tumors and STAT3. Upon binding of specific ligands, e.g., epidermal growth factor, interleukin -5 and -6 to the receptors, Janus kinases (JAKs) are activated, which in turn activates STAT3. Subsequently, it binds to the DNA in the nucleus resulting in the overexpression of genes involved in cell growth and metastasis, angiogenesis, and other cellular processes. STAT3 activation can also take place by mitogen-activated protein kinase (MAPK)-related signaling pathway. The activated STAT3 promotes carcinogenesis.[34] Another study indicated that STAT3 may act as tumor suppressor in different cancer types.[35] Natural products were used inhibitors to modulate the STAT3 signaling pathway.[36] Inhibitors were used to inhibit cell surface receptors (EGFR, human epidermal growth factor receptor 2 (HER2), platelet-derived growth factor receptor alpha (PDGFRA), Insulin Like Growth Factor 1 Receptor (IGFR), etc.) and downstream signaling including the STAT3 pathway. The steric hindrance by small phytochemical molecule is lower and can bind to DNA to inhibit the transcription factor activity of STAT3. A number of phytochemicals from diverse medicinal plants also have been reported to block STAT3 phosphorylation and nuclear translocation.[19] Natural products and many synthetic drugs as well may not be specific and selective enough to act on one molecular target.[37] Thereby binding to more than one target protein and affecting downstream signaling can occur. Deciphering the complexity of cellular mechanisms and signaling pathways related to cancer that are to be modulated by phytochemicals can be very challenging. Therefore, a cocktail of active phytochemicals for cancer therapy can be more effective. These mixtures of active phytochemicals can act on different checkpoints and as inhibitors of related signaling pathways.

# References

1. Li, C.Y., Mohd, T.N., and Li, S.C. (2015). A systematic review of integrated traditional Chinese and Western medicine for managing irritable bowel syndrome. *Am J Chin Med*. 43(3): 385–406. doi: 10.1142/S0192415X15500251

2. Arai, Y.C., Shimo, K., Inoue, M., *et al.* (2015). Integration of a Kampo medicine, Nijutsuto, and Western medical treatment in the treatment of long-term frozen shoulder refractory to Western medical treatment: a case series. *Evid Based Complementary Altern Med*. 20(2): 157–161. doi: 10.1177/2156587214568346

3. Fung, F.Y., and Linn, Y.C. (2015). Developing traditional Chinese medicine in the era of evidence-based medicine: current evidences and challenges. *Evid Based Complement Altern Med.* 2015: 425037. doi: 10.1155/2015/425037

4. Hsu, P.C., Tsai, Y.T., Lai, J.N., Wu, C.T., Lin, S.K., and Huang, C.Y. (2014). Integrating traditional Chinese medicine healthcare into diabetes care by reducing the risk of developing kidney failure among type 2 diabetic patients: a population-based case control study. *J Ethnopharmacol.* 156: 358–364. doi: 10.1016/j.jep.2014.08.029

5. Sun, Y. (2014). The role of Chinese medicine in clinical oncology. *Chin J Integr Med.* 20(1): 3–10. doi: 10.1007/s11655-013-1551-2

6. Lam, T.P., and Sun, K.S. (2013). Dilemma of integration with Western medicine — views of traditional Chinese medicine practitioners in a predominant Western medical setting. *Complement Ther Med.* 21(4): 300–305. doi: 10.1016/j.ctim.2013.04.003

7. Gouws, C., Steyn, D., Du Plessis, L., Steenekamp, J., and Hamman, J.H. (2012). Combination therapy of Western drugs and herbal medicines: recent advances in understanding interactions involving metabolism and efflux. *Expert Opin Drug Metab Toxicol.* 8(8): 973–84. doi: 10.1517/17425255.2012.691966

8. Xu, H., and Chen, K.J. (2010). Herb-drug interaction: an emerging issue of integrative medicine. *Chin J Integr Med.* 16(3): 195–196. doi: 10.1007/s11655-010-0195-z

9. Chan, E., Tan, M., Xin, J., Sudarsanam, S., and Johnson, D.E. (2010). Interactions between traditional Chinese medicines and Western therapeutics. *Curr Opin Drug Discov Devel.* 13(1): 50–65.

10. Seki, K., Chisaka, M., Eriguchi, M., *et al.* (2005, October). An attempt to integrate Western and Chinese medicine: rationale for applying Chinese medicine as chronotherapy against cancer. *Biomed Pharmacother.* 59(Suppl 1): S132–S140.

11. Dobos, G., and Tao, I. (2011). The model of Western integrative medicine: the role of Chinese medicine. *Chin J Integr Med.* 17: 11–20. doi: 10.1007/s11655-011-0601-x

12. Wong, R., Sagar, C.M., and Sagar, S.M. (2001). Integration of Chinese medicine into supportive cancer care. *Cancer Treat Rev.* 27(4): 235–246.

13. Dai, Y., Sun, L., and Qiang, W. (2018). A new strategy to uncover the anticancer mechanism of Chinese compound formula by integrating systems pharmacology and bioinformatics. *Evid Based Complement Altern Med.* 2018: 19. doi: 10.1155/2018/6707850

14. Yang, Y., Zhang, N., Li, K., Chen, J., Qiu, L., and Zhang, J. (2018). Integration of microRNA–mRNA profiles and pathway analysis of plant isoquinoline alkaloid berberine in SGC-7901 gastric cancers cells. *Drug Des Devel Ther.* 12: 393–408.

15. Tillhon, M., Guamán- Ortiz, L.M., Lombardi, P., and Scovassi, A.I. (2012). Berberine: new perspectives for old remedies. *Biochem Pharmacol.* 84(10): 1260–1267.

16. Yao, J., Kong, W., and Jiang, J. (2015). Learning from berberine: treating chronic diseases through multiple targets. *Sci China Life Sci.* 58(9): 854–859.

17. Ayati, S.H., Fazeli, B., Momtazi-Borojeni, A.A., Cicero, A.F.G., Pirro, M., and Sahebkar, A. (2017). Regulatory effects of berberine on microRNome in cancer and other conditions. *Crit Rev Oncol Hematol.* 116: 147–158.

18. Chang, W. (2017). Non-coding RNAs and berberine: a new mechanism of its anti-diabetic activities. *Eur J Pharmacol.* 795: 8–12.

19. Thomas, E., Mohamed, E.M.S., Elhaj, M., *et al.* (2017). Integration of phytochemicals and phytotherapy into cancer precision medicine. *Oncotarget.* 8(30): 50284–50304.

20. Lippert, T.H., Ruoff, H.J., and Volm, M. (2014). Could a revision of the current guidelines for cancer drug use improve the quality of cancer treatment? *Ther Clin Risk Manag.* 10: 69–72.

21. Mellor, H.R., and Callaghan, R. (2008). Resistance to chemotherapy in cancer: a complex and integrated cellular response. *Pharmacology.* 81: 275–300.

22. Walther, Z., and Sklar, J. (2011). Molecular tumor profiling for prediction of response to anticancer therapies. *Cancer J.* 17: 71–79.

23. Newman, D.J., and Cragg, G.M. (2007). Natural products as sources of new drugs over the last 25 years. *J Nat Prod.* 70: 461–477.

24. Kuete, V., and Efferth, T. (2010). Cameroonian medicinal plants: pharmacology and derived natural product. *Front Pharmacol.* 1: 123–130.

25. Wöll, S., Kim, S.H., and Efferth, T. (2013). Animal plant warfare and secondary metabolite evolution. *Nat Prod Bioprospect.* 3: 1–7.

26. Li, P.C., Lam, E., Roos, W.P., Zdzienicka, M.Z., Kaina, B., and Efferth, T. (2008). Artesunate derived from traditional Chinese medicine induces DNA damage and repair. *Cancer Res.* 68: 4347–4351.

27. Efferth, T., Konkimalla, V.B., Wang, Y.F., *et al.* (2008). Prediction of broad spectrum resistance of tumors towards anticancer drugs. *Clin Cancer Res.* 14: 2405–2412.

28. Wahl, O., Oswald, M., Tretzel, L., Herres, E., Arend, J., and Efferth, T. (2011). Inhibition of tumor angiogenesis by antibodies, synthetic small molecules and natural products. *Curr Med Chem.* 18: 3136–3155.

29. Saeed, M.E., Abdelgadir, H., Sugimoto, Y., Khalid, H.E., and Efferth, T. (2015). Cytotoxicity of 35 medicinal plants from Sudan towards sensitive and multidrug-resistant cancer cells. *J Ethnopharmacol.* 174: 644–655.

30. Saeed, M.E., Meyer, M., Hussein, A., and Efferth, T. (2016). Cytotoxicity of South-African medicinal plants towards sensitive and multidrug-resistant cancer cells. *J Ethnopharmacol.* 186: 209–223.

31. Omosa, L.K., Midiwo, J.O., Masila, V.M., *et al.* (2016). Cytotoxicity of 91 Kenyan indigenous medicinal plants towards human CCRF-CEM leukemia cells. *J Ethnopharmacol.* 179: 177–196.

32. Meyer-Hamme, G., Beckmann, K., Radtke, J., *et al.* (2013). A survey of Chinese medicinal herbal treatment for chemotherapy-induced oral mucositis. *Evid Based Complement Altern Med.* 2013: 284959.

33. Fong, S.Y., Efferth, T.H., and Zuo, Z. (2014). Modulation of the pharmacokinetics, therapeutic and adverse effects of NSAIDs by Chinese herbal medicines. *Expert Opin Drug Metab Toxicol.* 10: 1711–1739.

34. Resemann, H.K., Watson, C.J., and Lloyd-Lewis, B. (2014). The Stat3 paradox: a killer and an oncogene. *Mol Cell Endocrinol.* 382: 603–611.

35. Zhang, H.F., and Lai, R. (2014). STAT3 in cancer-friend or foe? *Cancers (Basel).* 6: 1408–1440.

36. Furtek, S.L., Backos, D.S., Matheson, C.J., and Reigan, P. (2016). Strategies and approaches of targeting STAT3 for cancer treatment. *ACS Chem Biol.* 11: 308–318.

37. Efferth, T., and Koch, E. (2011). Complex interactions between phytochemicals. The multi-target therapeutic concept of phytotherapy. *Curr Drug Targets.* 12: 122–132.

# 7

## CYTOTOXIC PLANT MOLECULES AND IMMUNOPHARMACOLOGY

Most of active anticancer phytochemicals display cytotoxic effects on cancer cells. The common mechanistic toxic action is through modulation of signaling pathways related to cell cycle arrest, differentiation, and cell growth processes. Aporphinoids are an important group of plant secondary metabolites from phytochemicals. Some of these compounds are used in traditional medicine for the treatment of various diseases for a long time. More than 500 aporphine alkaloids have been isolated from various plant families, and many of these compounds display potent cytotoxic activities.[1] An earlier study reported that the cytotoxic compounds include aporphinoids such as boldine, dicentrine, and oxo-, pro-, and dehydro-aporphines. Their mechanisms of action are not known, but the inhibitory activities toward polymerases and topoisomerases were reported.

# Role of the aporphinoids in the development of anticancer agents

Medicinal plants have been used for treatment diseases and healthcare in Asian countries and Western culture in last decade.[2] Diversity of phytochemicals and their metabolism in plants has provided a variety of lead structures in drug development and account for more than 50% of our current medicines. Research on natural compounds have been thriving in the field of anticancer drug development. In the United States, more than 60% of the approved anticancer drugs were from natural origin in the two decades.[3] A typical example is that of camptothecin, a monoterpenoid alkaloid, which was isolated from the Chinese ornamental tree *Camptotheca acuminata* in the sixties from which two derivatives irinotecan (a pro-drug) and less toxic topotecan than camptothecin itself were developed and are currently used as anticancer agents, for the treatment of colorectal and ovarian cancers in particular.

Taxols (paclitaxel and the semi-synthetic derivative docetaxel), *Vinca* alkaloids (vinblastine, vincristine, and the semi-synthetic derivative vinorelbine), and podophyllotoxins (the semi-synthetic derivatives: etoposide and teniposide) are among the most frequently used anticancer drugs.[4,5]

Alkaloids are abundant secondary metabolites in plants and represent one of the most widespread class of compounds with different pharmacological properties. Among alkaloids, the aporphinoids are a broad subgroup of benzylisoquinoline compounds, with more than 500 alkaloids known today. They are widely distributed in a large number of plant families including Annonaceae, Lauraceae, Monimiaceae, Menispermaceae, Hernandiaceae, and Ranunculaceae.[6] The chemistry, botanical sources, and pharmacological activities of aporphinoids, and the derivatives were described.[7–9] Aporphines are optically active, possessing either the R-(−) or S-(+).

## Cytotoxic and anticancer activities

The alkaloids and lignans were isolated from the trunk bark of *Hernandia nymphaeifolia* (Hernandiaceae) and were tested against four tumor cell lines *in vitro*, namely P388 leukemia, human mouth epidermoid KERATIN-forming tumor cell (KB)16 cells, A549 lung, and HT-29 colon cells.[10,11] The basic structure of apophine alkaloids is shown in Figure 7.1. Among the compounds evaluated, the two aporphines S-ovigerine, S-N-methylovigerine showed cytotoxic activities with IC50 values < 4 μM against the four cell lines. S-magnoflorine and Shernovine showed selective cytotoxicity against the P388 cell line with IC50 of 0.7 μM compared that of mithramycin, a reference anticancer agent, on one cell line or the other, such as S-N-hydroxyovigerine on KB16 cells and S-N-methylhernangerine and S-laurotetanine against P388 cells. The results showed that the noraporphine Shernovine exhibited more potent cytotoxic activity with IC50 of 0.7 μM on P-388 cells, 20 μM on HT-29 cells, and around 45 μM on KB16 and A549 cells than its methylated analog S-N-methylhernovine, which is inactive on all tested cells with IC50 > 153 μM.[10,11]

It is believed that the quaternization of the ring nitrogen of aporphines is involved in the cytotoxic action in cancer cells.[12] A number of benzylisoquinoline alkaloids, either isolated from plants indigenous to formosan or obtained by partial synthesis, were tested for their cytotoxic activities on a murine (L1210) and two leukemia cell lines: human cell type human leukemic lymphoblasts (CCRF-CEM) and cell type human promyelocytic leukemia (HL-60).[12] These compounds were shown to inhibit the incorporation of precursors into DNA, RNA, and proteins.

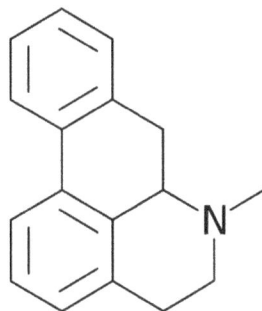

**Figure 7.1** Basic structure of aporphine.

The tertiary alkaloid dicentrine displayed cytotoxicity against the three cell lines with IC50 of 30 μM, while the quaternary derivative dicentrine MeI was inactive on the cell growth. One of the active aporphines tested was dicentrine (Figure 7.2), which exhibited strong inhibitory activities against the murine and human leukemic cells, with IC50 values around 3 μM and had considerable inhibitory effects on DNA, RNA, and proteins biosynthesis. However, the detailed mechanism of its inhibitory action of toward cell cycle and related signaling pathways remains unclear.[12]

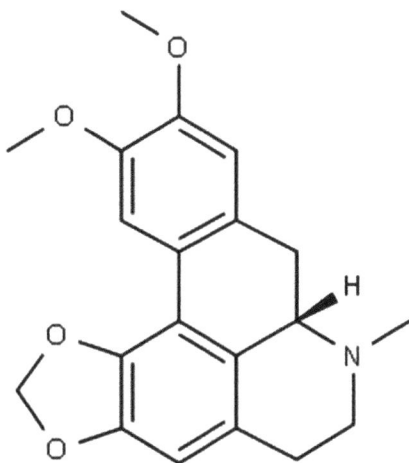

**Figure 7.2** Chemical structure of dicentrine.

## Isoquinoline cytotoxicity

The cytotoxic activities of some monomeric isoquinoline alkaloids including S-corydine and S-isocorydine did not exert inhibitory effects on human carcinoma of the nasopharynx,[13] and they are inactive *in vivo* against the Walker 256 tumor. Other study indicated that S-corydine was inactive on KB cells.[14] The results suggest that not all isoquinoline alkaloids show cytotoxic effects on cancer cells, yet the cytotoxicity relies on the structure–activity relationship and the substituents on the ring of the alkaloids.

## Cytotoxic actions of aporphines

Among aporphine alkaloids, *S*-dicentrine inhibited the mitogen-induced lymphocyte proliferation and the growth of IL-2-dependent cell type lymphocyte cytotoxic T lymphocyte (CTLL)2 line.[15] The cytotoxic (*in vitro*) and anti-tumor (*in vivo*) effects of *S*-dicentrine, which were isolated from *Lindera megaphylla* (Lauraceae), also exhibited cytotoxicity in the human hepatoma cell line HuH-7 through inhibition of DNA and RNA. The *in vitro* cytotoxicity study showed that *S*-dicentrine exhibited a cytotoxic effect in all tested cell lines with IC50 values ranging from 0.4 μM on the esophageal carcinoma cell line HCE-6 to up to 29 μM on the hepatoma cell line HA22T.[1,9].

The *in vivo* study revealed that dicentrine inhibited the growth of K562 cells in Severe combined immunodeficiency (SCID) mice. The results suggested that this compound exhibits cytostatic effects and antitumor activity.[16]

Among the aporphines tested, the following compounds were demonstrated with inhibitory effects on cell growth of cancer cell line (P3HR-1), kidney cell line (MK-2), and cell type Human epithelial type 2 (HEp-2) cells (HEP-2) cells[17]:

- Anonaine
- Actinodaphnine
- *N*-methylactinodaphnine (cassythicine)
- Dicentrine
- Glaucine
- Actinodaphnine

Other study showed that the extract of *Cassytha filiformis* (Lauraceae) exhibited *in vitro* cytotoxic effects through the cell cycle on HeLa, Mel-5, HL60 cancer cell lines and on cell type Fibroblasts cell line (NIH3T3) noncancer cells.[18] The results suggest cytotoxic agents inhibit the cell growth of cancer cells through inhibition of cell differentiation and the related signaling pathways, yet the cytotoxicity of alkaloids can vary in different types of cells. For example, actinodaphnine showed the highest activity against Mel-5 *in vitro* with (IC50 of 24.3 μM) and HL-60 with IC50 of 19.9 μM.[18]

The *in vitro* cytotoxicity activities of three *S*-alkaloids isolated from *C. filiformis* on *Trypanosoma brucei* demonstrated similar mode of action in DNA activity.

*S*-alkaloids interfere with the catalytic activity of topoisomerases.[19] Though *S*-bulbocapnine and *S*-dicentrine showed similar chemical structure, they differ in anti-tumor activity probably due to the presence of a hydroxyl group in the chemical structure.

Molecular modeling showed that dicentrine can take a planar conformation, whereas bulbocapnine cannot due to steric interactions between the substituents in the ring structure. The results suggested that the cytotoxicity of aporphinoids is associated with the steric hindrance in their ability to bind with DNA.[20]

Different aporphines isolated from *Stephania dinklagei* (Menispermaceae) showed different anti-tumor activities. Previous studies showed not all aporphines had cytotoxicity toward DNA.[20,21]

# The ethanol extract of *Stephania pierrei* (Menispermaceae)

The cytotoxic activities of isoquinoline alkaloids that were isolated from *Stephania pierrei* (Menispermaceae) against a large variety of mammalian cancer cell lines were evaluated.[22] The cytotoxicity of *S. pierrei* extracts was attributed to the presence of aporphine alkaloids. Those compounds lacking *N*-methylation or *N*-acetylation on the ring of aporphines did not exert inhibitory effect on cell growth. The results suggested that the methylenedioxy ring is involved in the mode of action with cell cycle. However, the detailed mechanism of actions of aporphine alkaloids remains sketchy.

The findings suggest not all cytotoxic agents can be worth further investigation for drug development, yet aporphines with methylenedioxy moiety may be administered as adjuvant for cancer therapy to reduce drug toxicity. An earlier study showed that *S*-glaucine isolated from plants from the *Corydalis* species (*C. bulbosa* and *C. pallida*) (Fumariaceae) exerted inhibitory effects against the Epstein–Barr virus early antigen activation induced by 12-O-tetradecanoylphorbol 13-acetate (TPA) in Raji cells.[23] It showed cytotoxicity in cells. The results suggested that *S*-glaucine demonstrated cancer chemopreventive action. The adjuvant effect was revealed in a study of *R*-roemerine, an aporphine isolated from the ethyl acetate extract of *Annona senegalensis* (Annonaceae).[24] This compound was tested on a series of human tumor cell lines and showed a moderate cytotoxicity but was found to enhance the cytotoxic response mediated by vinblastine in multidrug-resistant cell type human cervix carcinoma (KB-V1) cells.[1,23]

## Cytotoxicity of a spirostanol saponin

Natural products derived from plant sources have been used as source of potential therapeutic agents. *Rohdea chinensis* Baker (syn. *Tupistra chinensis*) (Convallariaceae) exists in Southwest China. Its dried rhizome is used in Chinese folk medicine to reduce carbuncles and to ameliorate pharyngitis.[25,26] Steroidal saponins were believed to be the main active ingredients in this plant. *R. chinensis* extracts inhibited cell proliferation and induced apoptosis in human A549 cells via mitochondria-dependent apoptotic pathways.[27]

Spirostanol saponins that was isolated from the rhizome of *R. chinensis* displayed potent anti-proliferative and anti-inflammatory activities.[28] Recent study showed that 5β-spirost-en-1β,3β-diol-1-*O*-α-L-rhamnopyranosyl-β-D-xylopyranosyl-3-*O*-α-L-rhamnopyranoside (SPD; Figure 7.3) induced apoptosis in HL-60 cells.[29] SPD also promoted apoptosis by induction of pro-death autophagy. The study suggests that phytochemical compounds with anticancer activity can exert cytotoxicity through apoptotic activity and disruption of the related signaling pathways in cell differentiation.

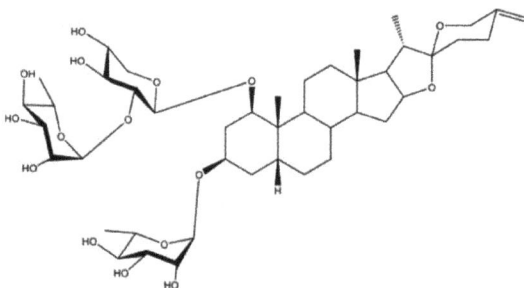

**Figure 7.3**  Chemical structure of 5β-spirost-25(27)-en-1β,3β-diol-1-*O*-α-L-rhamnopyranosyl-(1→2)-β-D-xylopyranosyl-3-*O*-α-L-rhamnopyranoside (SPD).

## Cytotoxic phytochemical compounds in cancer therapy

Traditional Chinese medicine (TCM) with anticancer properties has been used in folk medicine for the treatment of cancers. Most of the chemical components of herbal extracts contain various alkaloids, quinones, and triterpenoids. Some of these compounds showed cytotoxicity on cancer cells. But the details of cytotoxic mechanism of anticancer phytochemical compounds have not been fully understood. Cytotoxicity studies are useful initial step in determining the potential toxicity and the anticancer activity of chemical compounds in the active fractions of herbal extracts. Cellular toxicity studies would shed light on the deleterious effects on structures and functions common to human cells. This is important when considering the relationship between acute toxicity and cytotoxicity. The selectivity index is an important measure to identify active compounds with promising biological activity and anticancer properties. Table 7.1 shows various phytochemicals from herbal plants. Various bioassays and various types of cancer cell lines have to be used to assess cytotoxicity of herbal extracts. Most of anticancer compounds showed cytotoxicity on human cancer cell lines, through apoptosis induction and G0/G1 arrest in cells. Active compounds can promote signaling pathways related to apoptosis via the activation of extracellular signal–regulated kinase (ERK1/2) and c-Jun N-terminal kinase (JNK) pathway in Mitogen-activated protein kinase (MAPK) family, which in turn increased the expression of p53, thereby triggering the $G_0/G_1$ arrest through p53/p21/cyclin D1 signaling. Subsequently, JNK activation down-regulated the expression of the anti-apoptotic protein a complex structure of the cellular respiratory chain of mitochondria (Bcl-2), which caused the release of cytochrome $c$ to the cytosol and activated the cleavage of caspase cascade and poly (ADP-ribose) polymerase, thereby inducing apoptosis in cancer cells. In addition, anticancer compounds can inhibit the activation of a protein complex that controls transcription of DNA, cytokine production and cell survival (NF-κB) signaling by down-regulating the expression and attenuating the translocation to nucleus of NF-κB p65, by which the downstream p53, cyclin D1, Bcl-2, and caspase cascade can be modulated leading to apoptosis and $G_0/G_1$ arrest in cancer cells.[29,30] However, active phytochemicals may exert less cytotoxicity to normal cells.

A pharmacologically active phytochemical should bear smaller molecular size and cytotoxicity *in vitro* study that may facilitate the penetration of the active phytochemical into the system and induce apoptosis of cancer cells. Pharmaceutical drug development nowadays prefer small size natural products not only because it allows a more cost-effective synthetic route and a better pharmacological properties. Appendix III shows some of the common natural molecules from herbal medicines that can exhibit pharmacological effects. Large molecules, or biologics, are classified as macromolecules such as proteinous products having a limited therapeutic effect. In contrast to small molecule drugs, most large molecule drugs are complex that may not be able to enter cells readily. Small molecule can easily get inside the cells. It can affect other molecules, such as enzymes and gene expression proteins, and may cause cancer cells to die. Many targeted therapies are small molecule drugs or small molecule inhibitors.

**Table 7.1** Common cytotoxic phytochemical compounds

| Compound | Action | Reference |
|---|---|---|
| Hectochlorin | Significant cytotoxicity against colon, melanoma, ovarian, and renal cell lines | Tan[31], Marquez et al.[32], Ramaswamy et al.[33] |
| Lyngbyabellins | Significant cytotoxicity against various cell lines, including KB and H460 cancer cells | Tan[31], Yokokawa et al.[34] |
| Apratoxin A | Attenuating the fibroblast growth factor (FGF) signaling pathway | Tan[31] |
| Aurilides | Tumor cell-killing activity Cytotoxic to and to be particularly active against leukemia, renal, and prostate cancer cell lines | Tan[31], Han et al.[35] |
| Piplartine | Inhibition of the tumor proliferation rate (especially kidney) | Bezerra et al.[36] |
| Piperine | Cytotoxic activity toward tumor cell lines (especially liver) | Bezerra et al.[36] |
| Camptothecin (CPT) | Anticancer effect to colorectal and ovarian cancer | Stévigny et al.[1], Liu et al. [37] |
| Vinblastine | Antineoplastic agents (suppressed the rates of microtubule growth and shortening, and decreased the frequency of transitions from growth or pause to shortening, also called catastrophe) →Treatment for Hodgkin's lymphoma, nonsmall cell lung cancer, bladder cancer, brain cancer, and testicular cancer | Stévigny et al.[1], Dhamodharan et al.[38] |
| Vincristine | Acts by binding to tubulin and blocking metaphase in actively dividing cells | Stévigny et al.[1], Waterhouse et al.[39] |

| Compound | Action | Reference |
|---|---|---|
| Boldine | Free radical scavenger properties, cytotoxic effect, and induced apoptosis in breast cancer cells as indicated by a higher amount of lactate dehydrogenase released, membrane permeability, and DNA fragmentation | Stévigny *et al.*[1], Paydar *et al.*[40] |
| Actinodaphnine, cassythine, dicentrine | Interfere with the catalytic activity of topoisomerases, intercalating agent (dicentrine) cytotoxicity toward U87MG, activation of breast cancer type 1 susceptibility protein (BRCA1)-mediated DNA damage response, p53 signaling, G1/S and G2/M cell cycle regulation, and aryl hydrocarbon receptor | Stévigny *et al.*[1], Hoet *et al.*[18], Konkimalla and Efferth[41] |

# References

1. Stévigny, C., Bailly, C., and Quetin-Leclercq, J. (2005). Cytotoxic and antitumor potentialities of aporphinoid alkaloids. *Curr Med Chem Anticancer Agents.* 5: 173–182.
2. Phillipson, J.D. (2007). Phytochem pharmacognosy. *Phytochemistry.* 68(22–24): 2960–2972.
3. Takeuchi, M., Saito, Y., Goto, M., *et al.* (2018). Antiproliferative alkaloids from *Alangium longiflorum*, an endangered tropical plant species. *J Nat Prod.* 81(8): 1884–1891. doi: 10.1021/acs.jnatprod.8b00411
4. Ferrari, J., Terreaux, C., Sahpaz, S., Msonthi, J.D., Wolfender, J.L., and Hostettmann, K. (2000). Benzophenone glycosides from *Gnidia onvolucrata*. *Phytochemistry.* 54(8): 883–889.
5. Aouey, B., Samet, A.M., Fetoui, H., Simmonds, M.S.J., and Bouaziz, M. (2016). Anti-oxidant, anti-inflammatory, analgesic and antipyretic activities of grapevine leaf extract (*Vitis vinifera*) in mice and identification of its active constituents by LC-MS/MS analyses. *Biomed Pharmacother.* 84: 1088–1098. doi: 10.1016/j.biopha.2016.10.033
6. Angerhofer, C.K., Guinaudeau, H., Wongpanich, V., Pezzuto, J., and Cordell, G.A. (1999). Antiplasmodial and cytotoxic activity of natural bisbenzylisoquinoline alkaloids. *J Nat Prod.* 62(1): 59–66.
7. Guinaudeau, H., Lin, L.Z., Ruangrungsi, N., and Cordell, G.A. (1993). Bisbenzylisoquinoline alkaloids from *Cyclea barbata*. *J Nat Prod.* 56(11): 1989–1992.
8. Cuéllar, M.J., Giner, R.M., Recio, M.C., Máñez, S., and Ríos, J.L. (2001). Topical anti-inflammatory activity of some Asian medicinal plants used in dermatological disorders. *Fitoterapia.* 72(3): 221–229.

9. Cordell, G.A. (2000), Biodiversity and drug discovery—a symbiotic relationship. *Phytochem.* 55(6): 463–480.

10. Chen, J.J., Ishikawa, T., Duh, C.Y., Tsai, I.L., and Chen, I.S. (1996). New dimeric aporphine alkaloids and cytotoxic constituents of *Hernandia nymphaeifolia*. *Planta Med.* 62: 528–533.

11. Chen, I.S., Chen, J.J., Duh, C.Y., Tsai, I.L., and Chang, C.T. (1997). New aporphine alkaloids and cytotoxic constituents of *Hernandia nymphaeifolia*. *Planta Med.* 63: 154–157.

12. Tseng, C.H., Tzeng, C.C., Hsu, C.Y., Cheng, C.M., Yang, C.N., and Chen, Y.L. (2015). Discovery of 3-phenylquinolinylchalcone derivatives as potent and selective anticancer agents against breast cancers. *Eur J Med Chem.* 97: 306–319. doi: 10.1016/j.ejmech

13. Wright, C.W., Marshall, S.J., Russell, P.F., *et al.* (2000). In vitro antiplasmodial, antiamoebic, and cytotoxic activities of some monomeric isoquinoline alkaloids. *J Nat Prod.* 63: 1638–1640.

14. Kupchan, S.M., and Altland, H.W. (1973). Structural requirements for tumor-inhibitory activity among benzylisoquinoline alkaloids and related synthetic compounds. *J Med Chem.* 16: 913–917.

15. Endo, T., Samokhvalov, V., Darwesh, A.M., *et al.* (2018). DHA and 19,20-EDP induce lysosomal-proteolytic-dependent cytotoxicity through de novo ceramide production in H9c2 cells with a glycolytic profile. *Cell Death Discov.* 20: 15–29. doi: 10.1038/s41420-018-0090-1

16. Huang, R.L., Chen, C.C., Huang, Y.L., *et al.* (1998). Anti-tumor effects of d-dicentrine from the root of *Lindera megaphylla*. *Planta Med.* 64: 212–215.

17. Huang, C.Y., Hsu, T.C., Kuo, W.W., *et al.* (2015). The root extract of *Gentiana macrophylla* Pall. Alleviates cardiac apoptosis in lupus prone mice. *PLoS ONE.* 10(5): e0127440. doi: 10.1371/journal.pone.0127440

18. Hoet, S., Stévigny, C., Block, S., *et al.* (2004). Alkaloids from *Cassytha filiformis* and related aporphines: antitrypanosomal activity, cytotoxicity, and interaction with DNA and topoisomerases. *Planta Med.* 70(5): 407–413.

19. Wu, Y.C., Liou, Y.F., Lu, S.T., Chen, C.H., Chang, J.J., and Lee, K.H. (1989). Cytotoxicity of isoquinoline alkaloids and their N-oxides. *Planta Med.* 55(2): 163–165.

20. Woo, S.H., Sun, N.J., Cassady, J.M., and Snapka, R.M. (1999). Topoisomerase II inhibition by aporphine alkaloids. *Biochem Pharmacol.* 57: 1141–1145.

21. Zhou, B.N., Johnson, R.K., Mattern, M.R., *et al.* (2000). Use of COMPARE analysis to discover new natural product drugs: isolation of camptothecin and 9-methoxy-camptothecin from a new source. *J Nat Prod.* 63(2): 217–221.

22. Likhitwitayawuid, K., Angerhofer, C.K., Chai, H., Pezzuto, J.M., Cordell, G.A., and Ruangrungsi, N. (1993). Cytotoxic and antimalarial alkaloids from the tubers of *Stephania pierrei*. *J Nat Prod.* 56: 1468–1478.

23. Ito, C., Itoigawa, M., Tokuda, H., Kuchide, M., Nishino, H., and Furukawa, H. (2001). Chemopreventive activity of isoquinoline alkaloids from Corydalis plants. *Planta Med.* 67: 473–475.

24. You, M., Wickramaratne, D.B.M., Silva, G.L., *et al.* (1995). (-)-Roemerine, an aporphine alkaloid from *Annona senegalensis* that reverses the multidrug-resistance phenotype with cultured cells. *J Nat Prod.* 58: 598–604.

25. Xiaomin, Y., Limin, X., Huanga, Y., Wang, Y., and He, X. (2018). Apoptosis and prodeath autophagy induced by a spirostanol saponin isolated from *Rohdea chinensis*

(Baker) N. Tanaka (synonym *Tupistra chinensis* Baker) on HL-60 cells. *Phytomedicine.* 42: 83–89. doi: 10.1016/j.phymed.2018.03.030

26. Xiang, L., Wang, Y., Yi, X., Zheng, G., and He, X. (2016). Bioactive spirostanol saponins from the rhizome of *Tupistra chinensis. Steroids.* 108: 39–46.

27. Huang, W., Zhang, H., Zou, K., *et al.* (2012). Total saponins of *Tupistra chinensis* induce apoptosis in A549 cells. *Neoplasma.* 59: 613–621.

28. Xiang, L., Wang, Y., Yi, X., and He, X. (2016). Antiproliferative and anti-inflammatory furostanol saponins from the rhizomes of *Tupistra chinensis. Steroids.* 116: 28–37.

29. Xiang, L., Wang, Y., Yi, X., Feng, J., and He, X. (2016). Furospirostanol and spirostanol saponins from the rhizome of *Tupistra chinensis* and their cytotoxic and anti-inflammatory activities. *Tetrahedron.* 72: 134–141.

30. Mbaveng, A.T., Fotso, G.W., Ngnintedo, D., *et al.* (2018). Cytotoxicity of epunctanone and four other phytochemicals isolated from the medicinal plants *Garcinia epunctata* and *Ptycholobium contortum* towards multi-factorial drug resistant cancer cells. *Phytomedicine.* 48: 112–119. doi: 10.1016/j.phymed.2017.12.016

31. Tan, L.T. (2007). Bioactive natural products from marine cyanobacteria for drug discovery. *Phytochemistry.* 68(7): 954–979.

32. Marquez, B.L., Watts, K.S., Yokochi, A., *et al.* (2002). Structure and absolute stereochemistry of hectochlorin, a potent stimulator of actin assembly. *J Nat Prod.* 65: 866–871.

33. Ramaswamy, A.V., Sorrels, C.M., and Gerwick, W.H. (2007). Cloning and biochemical characterization of the hectochlorin biosynthetic gene cluster from the marine cyanobacterium *Lyngbya majuscula. J Nat Prod.* 70(12): 1977–1986.

34. Yokokawa, F., Sameshima, H., Katagiri, D., Aoyama, T., and Shioiri, T. (2002). Total syntheses of lyngbyabellins A and B, potent cytotoxic lipopeptides from the marine cyanobacterium *Lyngbya majuscule. Tetrahedron.* 58(46): 9445–9458.

35. Han, B., Gross, H., Goeger, D.E., Mooberry, S.L., and Gerwick, W.H. (2006). Aurilides B and C, cancer cell toxins from a Papua New Guinea collection of the marine cyanobacterium *Lyngbya majuscula. J Nat Prod.* 69(4): 572–575.

36. Bezerra, D.P., Castro, F.O., Alves, A.P.N.N., Pessoa, C., Moraes, M.O., and Silveira, E.R. (2006). In vivo growth-inhibition of Sarcoma 180 by piplartine and piperine, two alkaloid amides from Piper. *Braz J Med Biol Res.* 39(6): 801–807.

37. Liu, L.F., Desai, S.D., Li, T.K., Mao, Y., Sun, M., and Sim, S.P. (2000). Mechanism of action of camptothecin. *Ann N Y Acad Sci.* 922: 1–10.

38. Dhamodharan, R., Jordan, M.A., Thrower, D., Wilson, L., and Wadsworth, P. (1995). Vinblastine suppresses dynamics of individual microtubules in living interphase cells. *Mol Biol Cell.* 6(9): 1215–1229.

39. Waterhouse, D.N., Madden, T.D., Cullis, P.R., Bally, M.B., Mayer, L.D., and Webb, M.S. (2005). Preparation, characterization, and biological analysis of liposomal formulations of vincristine. *Methods Enzymol.* 391: 40–57.

40. Paydar, M., Kamalidehghan, B., Wong, Y.L., Wong, W.F., Looi, C.Y., and Mustafa, M.R. (2014). Evaluation of cytotoxic and chemotherapeutic properties of boldine in breast cancer using in vitro and in vivo models. *Drug Des Devel Ther.* 8: 719–733.

41. Konkimalla, V.B., and Efferth, T. (2010). Inhibition of epidermal growth factor receptor over-expressing cancer cells by the aphorphine-type isoquinoline alkaloid, dicentrine. *Biochem Pharmacol.* 79(8): 1092–1099.

# POTENTIAL BENEFICIAL EFFECTS
# OF PLANT PRODUCTS

Although various herbal products are widely consumed in China and elsewhere, the chemical and pharmaceutical mechanism of actions of phytochemicals underpinning the healthcare benefits is poorly understood. This has hampered the process of herbal product development. Moreover, safety issues associated with the consumption of herbal products have recently aroused public awareness and extensive research in herbal medicine. Some herbal supplements and teas such as *Lithospermum officinale* have been reported to contain pyrrolizidine alkaloids, which may lead to hepatotoxicity following the long-term consumption.[1,2] It is important to provide evidence-based and scientific information on the herbal medicine with traditional healthcare uses. Due to changes in food and drug safety worldwide, individuals are increasingly using natural and traditional herbal remedies. This has boosted the demand for herbal products throughout the world.[3] The market for beverages including herbal teas has experienced a boom period over the past decade, with an annual increase in consumption of more than 20% to reach 80 million tons in 2015.[4] Numerous food industries and pharmaceutical research are involved in the development and promotion of new products based on Traditional Chinese Medicine (TCM).[5]

# Evidence-based validation of herbal medicine for healthcare products

Excess fat accumulation in the torso can result in health problems such as diabetes, hypertension, and dyslipidemia. Per World Health Organization, large population of the world is suffering from obesity and obesity-related disorders. Intensive efforts are focused on finding effective anti-obesity drugs and alternative medicine. However, drug development for treatment of diseases such as obesity is tedious. Alternative medicine for the prevention and treatment of diseases shows promise. Healthcare products based on TCM has a beneficial effect over conventional products due to therapeutic benefits in addition to nutritional supplement with improved safety issues. Many plants and plant-derived products showed beneficial effects on the body. The phytochemical compounds exert their effect through multiple mechanism of actions on biochemical process and physiological activity.[6]

A recent study showed that the fruit rind of *Garcinia gummi-gutta*, commonly known as *Garcinia cambogia* (syn.), is extensively used traditionally as a flavorant in fish curries due to its sharp sour taste. Additional uses include its use as a digestive and a traditional remedy to treat bowel complaints, intestinal parasites, and rheumatism.[7] This small size fruit is used in a weight-loss supplement. Studies have shown that the extracts and the active (–)-hydroxycitric acid (HCA) exhibited anti-obesity activity including reduced food intake and body fat gain by regulating the serotonin levels to modulate fat oxidation and de novo lipogenesis. HCA is a potent inhibitor of adenosine triphosphate-citrate lyase, for the conversion process of citrate to acetyl-coenzyme A, which plays a key role in fatty acid, cholesterol, and triglyceride syntheses. The crude extract from the plant also exerted hypolipidemic, antidiabetic, anti-inflammatory, anticancer, and hepatoprotective activities *in vitro* and *in vivo*. Phytochemical studies of the plant parts revealed the presence of mainly xanthones (e.g., carbogiol) and benzophenones (e.g., garcinol) and organic acids (e.g., HCA). Currently, a number of dietary supplements that contain cambogia and HCA for weight management are sold although the possible toxicity associated with the long-term use of these supplements remains unclear. However, the active components in formulations of the healthcare products need to be identified and evaluated.

# Analysis of bioactivity health of dietary flavonoids in healthcare products

Plant secondary metabolites can be used as protective agents in dietary products. In particular, the involvement of flavonoids and related compounds has become a major topic in human nutrition research. Evidence from epidemiological studies suggested the protective effects of various (poly)phenol-rich foods against several chronic diseases, including neurodegeneration, cancer, and cardiovascular diseases.[8] In recent years, the use of High Performance Liquid Chromatography-Mass Spectrometry (HPLC–MS) for the analysis of flavonoids and related compounds in foods and biological samples provides evidence on the (poly)phenol bioavailability. These advancements have led to improvements in identifying food composition and to establish metabolomic databases. Efforts to set up standard operation procedures for sample analysis and identification of active compounds improve the quantitative analysis of (poly)phenol metabolites and catabolites. Application of the protocols with appropriate model test systems helps to uncover potential mechanisms of actions of active compounds.

# Healthcare products with sulfur-containing compounds from *Allium cepa*

Diabetes mellitus (DM) is a common disease and its prevalence is increasing worldwide. Although antidiabetic drugs are known to ameliorate the symptoms of diabetes, they may cause adverse effects. Therefore, alternative medicine including TCM is used to supplement the treatment method. A previous study indicated that the efficacy of *Allium cepa* was an effective ingredient in dietary supplement. *A. cepa*, a spice plant, is commonly known as onion and belongs to the family Liliaceae. Since ancient times, it has been used traditionally for the treatment of different diseases through regulation of hypoglycemic activity. Sulfur compounds including *S*-methylcysteine and flavonoids such as quercetin are mainly responsible for the hypoglycemic activity of *A. cepa*.[9] *S*-methylcysteine and flavonoids can decrease the levels of blood glucose, serum lipids, oxidative stress, and lipid peroxidation, as well as increasing antioxidant enzyme activity and insulin secretion.[9] Extracts of onion have been shown to have hypoglycemic and hypolipidemic effects by modulating the activities of liver hexokinase, glucose 6-phosphatase, and Hydroxy-3-methyl-glutaryl (HMG) coenzyme-A reductase.[10] The study showed that patients with diabetes consumed slices of *A. cepa*, exhibited sufficient hypoglycemic activity. However, detail of *A. cepa* activity and its active components is lacking. The therapeutic benefits of *A. cepa* consumption should be characterized to provide supporting evidence on the consumption of dietary onion that could lower blood glucose levels and therefore to reduce health risk factors associated with diabetes.

# A nutraceutical approach with red grapes against diseases

Polyphenols are one of the major ingredients present in red grapes and in healthcare products. Polyphenols are associated with the prevention of diseases caused through ameliorating oxidative stress. The health benefits of polyphenols in grapes against diseases are known.[11] Health products are developed as nutraceuticals. Grape polyphenols displayed modulating effects on regulation of endothelial function with antioxidant capacity, which can reduce oxidation of low density of lipoprotein. Oxidized low-density lipoprotein (Ox-LDL) particles play a key role in the pathogenesis of atherosclerosis. The lipid-lowering properties and antioxidants of the grape seed can be beneficial in atherosclerosis prevention.[12] Lipid profiles and Ox-LDL in test subjects were measured at the beginning and the end of the study period. The results showed that red grape seed extract consumption reduced the level of total cholesterol, LDL cholesterol (LDL-C), and Ox-LDL. While triglyceride and very low-density lipoprotein cholesterol were decreased, high-density lipoprotein cholesterol was increased. The results suggested that red grape seed contained anti-oxidant effects on lipid profile, and it consequently decreased the risk of atherosclerosis and cardiovascular disorders.

# Benefits of phenolic compounds

Blueberries are rich in phenolic compounds with high antioxidant capacity. Experimental evidence suggested that blueberries and the phenolic compounds were effective anticancer agents, which were prepared both in the form of functional foods and as nutritional supplements.[13]

Some of the mechanism of actions have been shown to prevent carcinogenesis include inhibition of the production of pro-inflammatory molecules and oxidative stress. DNA damage can be modulated, and inhibition of cancer cell proliferation was increased. Clinical evidence supports nutritional supplements-containing blueberries can be used as anticancer agents. The nutritional properties of plants including medicinal plants vary, and the nutrient bioavailability are scarce although such information is required to evaluate phytochemicals as a healthcare product. In a previous study, extracts of marine algae wakame (*Undaria pinnatifida*) and nori (*Porphyra purpurea*) could lower the LDL-C level in rats, and intestinal leucine aminopeptidase activity was higher in rats fed with dietary supplements containing the extracts. However, the mechanistic actions of the extract remained unclear.[14,15]

## Therapeutic and health products with active plant extracts

Dietary supplements with TCM are popular among cancer patients due to its health benefits. An early study reported that double-blind, placebo-controlled randomized clinical trials (RCTs) of non-herbal dietary supplements (NHDS) and vitamins for evidence that prostate-specific antigen (PSA) levels were reduced in patients with Pachyonychia Congenit (PC).[16] Other supplements that contained isoflavones (genistein, daidzein, and glycitein), minerals (Se), or vitamins (vitamin D) or a combination of antioxidants, bioflavonoids, carotenoids, lycopenes, minerals (Se, Zn, Cu, and Mg), phytoestrogens, phytosterols, vitamins (B2, B6, B9, B12, C, and E), and other substances (CoQ10 and *n*-acetyl-l cysteine) were tested. Two RCTs reported that a combination of antioxidants, isoflavones, lycopenes, minerals, plant estrogens, and vitamins significantly decreased PSA levels compared with placebo. The results suggested that dietary supplements with specific remedies were effective for cancer patients, yet even for these supplements, additional clinical evidence is necessary before firm recommendations would be justified.

Metabolism of phytochemical compounds could produce oxidant metabolites with toxic effect when they are bioaccumulated in the body resulting in oxidative stress and diseases. Phytochemical compounds with antioxidative activity can reduce the oxidative stress through either reducing the formation of oxidants or removing free radical intermediates leading to prevention of oxidative damage. Different sources of naturally occurring antioxidants including those with proven activities from medicinal plants are available. Some of the antioxidants from plants and vegetables, such as vitamins A, C, and E and polyphenols, have been used in dietary supplements.[17] It was reported that regular consumption of dietary supplements with anti-oxidants was useful for the control of chronic diseases. More specifically, fruits and vegetables have been shown to exert a protective effect.

Fruit pods contain various beneficial compounds that were shown to have anti-oxidative activities.[18] The edible parts of fruits were used as a source of pharmaceutical and nutraceutical products. It was reported that most fruit pods contain polyphenolic components that can promote antioxidant effects on human health. Moreover, the polyphenolic ingredients displayed anti-inflammatory, antibacterial, and chemopreventive effects. Besides polyphenolics, other compounds such as xanthones, carotenoids, and saponins also exhibited health benefits. The extracts of fruit pods were used in pharmaceutical products. Fruit pods or pericarp of *Garcinia mangostana, Ceratonia siliqua, Moringa oleifera, Acacia nilotica, Sapindus rarak*, and *Prosopis cineraria* were the common source for manufacturing of pharmaceutic products. Although the mechanistic actions of fruit pod extracts are not fully understood, the fruit pods of medicinal plants might be useful sources of nutraceutical and other pharmaceutical components. Rosemary extracts that contain phenolic compounds are effective antioxidants with other beneficial effects including antimicrobial, antiviral, anti-inflammatory, and anticarcinogenic activities[19] and are also known to be an effective chemopreventive agent.[19,20] Therefore, this species contains the compounds with health benefits and was applied in the food industry, yet the mechanism of actions of the extracts remains unclear. The biological activity and safety of therapeutic and health products including herbal dietary supplements should be characterized and assured prior to use. The results can provide insights into development of new cancer chemopreventive compounds based on plant extracts, and the findings would enhance complementary treatments with drugs. It is advantageous to develop a generic method for the multitargeted screening of biomarkers, which aims at characterizing plant species in pharmaceutical supplements.

## Functional food with bioactive compounds

Seaweed biomass has been used for various intents in food including sta-bilizing agents. Biorefineries with seaweed as feedstock and food prod-ucts attract worldwide interest and include high value-added products.[21] Studies on bioactive compounds in seaweed usually focused on just a few species and compounds. An early review reported worldwide research on bioactive compounds, mainly of nine genera or species of seaweed, which are available in European temperate Atlantic waters, that is, *Laminaria* sp., *Fucus* sp., *Ascophyllum nodosum*, *Chondrus crispus*, *Porphyra* sp., *Ulva* sp., *Sargassum* sp., Gracilaria sp., and *Palmaria palmata*. *U. pinnatifida* is one of the most commonly investigated and available species globally. In addition, scientific experiments performed on seaweed used as animal feed suggested that seaweed provides a good source of bioactive compounds and health products.

## Flavonoids and phenolics in health products

The common source of functional phytochemicals is not only found in TCM but also in fruits and vegetables. Berries contain vitamin C and are a rich source of phytochemicals, especially anthocyanins and phenolic compounds, including ellagitannins, flavan-3-ols, procyanidins, flavonols, and hydroxybenzoate derivatives.[22] The study showed involvement of the colonic microflora in catabolizing dietary flavonoids that pass from the small to the large intestine. The results suggest the role of the resultant phenolic acids and the use of flavonoids in health products.

The *in vitro* and *in vivo* study of bioactivities of these polyphenol metabolites and catabolites reflected the protective effects of dietary poly-phenols in the digestive tract.[23]

As the epidemic of obesity, diabetes, and hypertension continues to grow among young adults, the population at risk for atherosclerotic coronary heart disease is increasing. LDL is the major atherogenic lipo-protein. Clinical data that showed dietary supplements with statins dis-played efficacy of lowering LDL-C for reducing coronary heart disease risk.[24] Although statins are relatively safe, there are still a number of patients who cannot tolerate them. The results suggested that patients preferred alternatives to statin therapy. Although a number of dietary supplements and functional foods could reduce LDL-C levels, they need more systematic data from the human trial. Yet the evidence in support of dietary supplements and their LDL-C-lowering effects showed promise. However, dietary supplements with various compositions of phyto-chemicals were not found to lower LDL-C.

# Flavanols in *Allium* species

Onion (*A. cepa* L.) is in the Liliaceae family and is a species that are abundant across a wide range of latitudes and altitudes in Europe, Asia, North America, and Africa. World onion production has increased by at least 25% over the past 10 years, with current production being around 44 million ton making it the second most important agricultural pro-duce after tomatoes.[25] Because of their easy storage and health benefits, onions are one of the most popular vegetables worldwide. Onion extracts and the active ingredients are often used in many food products and healthcare supplements. Onion consumption is increasing significantly, particularly in the United States due to the awareness of the health ben-efits of the flavonoids and the alk(en)yl cysteine sulfoxides (ACSOs) in onions. Two flavonoid subgroups are found in onion, the anthocyanins, which impart a purple color in onions, and flavanols such as quercetin and its derivatives, which are responsible for the yellow and brown skins of many other varieties. The ACSOs are the flavor precursors, which can generate the characteristic odor through enzymatic reactions and taste of onion. The enzymatic products are a complex mixture of compounds, which include thiosulfinates, thiosulfonates, mono-, di- and tri-sulfides. Like other anthocyanin and flavanol compounds, these groups of com-pounds in onion have been reported to have a multi-array of health benefits including anticarcinogenic properties, antiplatelet activity, anti-thrombotic activity, antiasthmatic, and antibiotic effects. Garlic (*Allium sativum* L.) showed similar health benefits. Until now, the lipid-lowering and anti-obesity functions of garlic oil and onion oil are not clear. A recent study reported the effects of garlic oil and onion oil on serum lipid levels in hyperlipidemia model rats.[26] The results showed that both extracts contained a complex mixture of compounds that could prevent hyper-lipidemia in the rat. The extracts could be developed through a dietary approach. The results provide supporting evidence on the health benefits of garlic and onion.

# References

1. Yao, F., Yang, J., Cunningham, A., (2018). A billion cups: the diversity, traditional uses, safety issues and potential of Chinese herbal teas. *J Ethnopharmacol.* 222: 217–228.
2. Santayana, M.P.D., Blanco, E., and Morales, R. (2005). Plants known as *t´e* in Spain: an ethno-pharmaco-botanical review. *J Ethnopharmacol.* 98: 1–19.
3. Siegrist, M., Shi, J., Giusto, A., and Hartmann, C. (2015). Worlds apart. Consumer acceptance of functional foods and beverages in Germany and China Appetite. *Appetite.* 92(2015): 87–93
4. Xie, P.J., Huang, L.X., Zhang, C.H., You, F., Zhang, Y.L., and Sun, G.G. (2014). Determination and analysis of chemical compositions on dandelion tea and leaves. *Sci Technol Food Ind.* 15: 346–351.
5. Liu, Y.L., Ahmed, S., and Long, C.L. (2013). Ethnobotanical survey of cooling herbal drinks from southern China. *J Ethnobiol Ethnomed.* 9: 82–87.
6. Navarro, V.J., Khan, I., Bjornsson, E., Seeff, B.L., Serrano, J., and Hoofnagle, H.J. (2017). Liver injury from herbal and dietary supplements. *Hepatology.* 65(1): 363–373.
7. Semwal, R.B., Semwal, D.K., Vermaak, I., and Viljoen, A. (2015). A comprehensive scientific overview of *Garcinia cambogia*. *Fitoterapia.* 102: 134–148. doi: 10.1016/j.fitote.2015.02.012.
8. Rodriguez-Mateos, A., Vauzour, D., Krueger, C.G., *et al.* (2014). Bioavailability, bioactivity and impact on health of dietary flavonoids and related compounds: an update. *Arch Toxicol.* (10): 1803–1853. doi: 10.1007/s00204-014-1330-7.
9. Akash M.S., Rehman K., and Chen S. (2014, October 30). Spice plant *Allium cepa*: dietary supplement for treatment of type 2 diabetes mellitus. *Nutrition.* 2014(10): 1128–1137. doi: 10.1016/j.nut.2014.02.011. Epub 2014 Mar 2.
10. Zeng, Y., Li, Y., Yang, J., *et al.* (2017). Therapeutic role of functional components in *Alliums* for preventive chronic disease in human being. *Evid Based Complement Alternat Med.* 2017. 9402849. doi: 10.1155/2017/9402849. Epub 2017 Feb 5.
11. Gollucke A.P., Peres R.C., Odair A Jr., and Ribeiro D.A. (2013, December 5). Polyphenols: a nutraceutical approach against diseases. *Recent Pat Food Nutr Agric.* 2013 (3): 214–219.
12. Razavi, S.M., Gholamin, S., Eskandari,A., *et al.* (2013). Red grape seed extract improves lipid profiles and decreases oxidized low-density lipoprotein in patients with mild hyperlipidemia. *J Med Food.* 16(3): 255–258. doi: 10.1089/jmf.2012.2408.
13. Johnson, S.A., and Arjmandi, B.H. (2013). Evidence for anti-cancer properties of blueberries: a mini-review. *Anticancer Agents Med Chem.* 13(8): 1142–1148.
14. Taboada, M.C., Millán, R., and Miguez, M.I. (2013). Nutritional value of the marine algae wakame (*Undaria pinnatifida*) and nori (*Porphyra purpurea*) as food supplements. *J Appl Phycol.* 25(5): 1271–1276.
15. Taboada, M.C., Millan, R., and Miguez, I. (2013). Evaluation of marine algae *Undaria pinnatifida* and *Porphyra purpurea* as a food supplement: Composition, nutritional value and effect of intake on intestinal, hepatic and renal enzyme activities in rats. *J Sci Food Agric.* 93(8): 1863–1868. doi: 10.1002/jsfa.5981.
16. Posadzki, P., Lee, M.S., Onakpoya, I., Lee, H.W., Ko, B.S., and Ernst, E. (2013). Dietary supplements and prostate cancer: a systematic review of double-blind, placebo-controlled randomised clinical trials. *Maturitas.* 2013. 75(2): 125–130. doi: 10.1016/j.maturitas.2013.03.006.

17. Landete, J.M. (2013). Dietary intake of natural antioxidants: vitamins and polyphenols. *Crit Rev Food Sci Nutr.* 53(7): 706–721. doi: 10.1080/10408398.2011.555018.
18. Karim, A.A., Azlan, A., Karim, A.A., and Azlan, A. (2012). Fruit pod extracts as a source of nutraceuticals and pharmaceuticals. *Molecules.* 10, 17(10): 11931–11946. doi: 10.3390/molecules171011931.
19. Aherne, S.A., Kerry, J.P., and O'Brien, N.M. (2007). Effects of plant extracts on antioxidant status and oxidant-induced stress in Caco-2 cells. *Br J Nutr.* 97(2): 321–328.
20. Daly, T., Jiwan, M.A., O'Brien, N.M., and Aherne, S.A. (2010). Carotenoid content of commonly consumed herbs and assessment of their bioaccessibility using an in vitro digestion model. *Plant Foods Hum Nutr.* 65(2): 164–169. doi: 10.1007/s11130-010-0167-3.
21. LøvstadHoldt, S., and Stefan, K.S. (2011). Bioactive compounds in seaweed: functional food applications and legislation. *J Appl Phycol.* 23(3): 543–597.
22. Aedin, C. (2018). Berry anthocyanin intake and cardiovascular health. *Mol Aspects Med.* 61: 76–82.
23. Del Rio, D., Borges, G., and Crozier, A. (2010). Berry flavonoids and phenolics: bioavailability and evidence of protective effects. *Br J Nutr.* 104(Suppl 3): S67–S90. doi: 10.1017/S0007114510003958.
24. Nijjar, P.S., Burke, F.M., Bloesch, A., and Rader, D.J. (2010). Role of dietary supplements in lowering low-density lipoprotein cholesterol: a review. *J Clin Lipidol.* (4): 248–258. doi: 10.1016/j.jacl.2010.07.001.
25. Griffiths, G., Trueman, L., Crowther, T., Thomas, B., and Smith, B. (2002). Onions— a global benefit to health. *Phytother Res.* 16(7): 603–615.
26. Yang, C., Li, L., Yang, L., Lu, H., Wang, S., and Sun, G. (2018). Anti-obesity and Hypolipidemic effects of garlic oil and onion oil in rats fed a high-fat diet. *Nutr Metab.* 15: 43–51. doi: 10.1186/s12986-018-0275-x.

# ADVERSE DRUG REACTIONS

Many prescribed drugs and established medicine can produce adverse drug reactions (ADRs) that may cause health risks. ADRs can be associated with loss seizures, convulsions, and health problems. In a recent study, the correlation between human ADR and signaling process in animal studies showed drug-induced ADR leading to loss of consciousness and convulsions.[1-2] Of 393 medicines taken, 101 (25.7%) showed loss of consciousness and 105 (26.7%) showed seizures or convulsions and/ or affecting the central nervous system. The study reported that the animal toxicity concordance ratio with syncope/loss of consciousness and seizures/convulsions was 4.0% (4 of 101) and 23.8% (25 of 105), respectively. The underlying cases of syncope/loss of consciousness was attributed to hypotension, arrhythmia, hypoglycemia, or toxic metabolites was 16.8%, 5.0%, 4.0%, or 4.0%, respectively.[1] However, the mechanism of seizures/ convulsions for the remaining 101 medicines remained unclear. The results suggest that metabolism of drugs would produce toxicity upon long-term intake of drugs, yet individual responses to drugs vary. An evaluation of drug safety in humans should be conducted to ameliorate drug toxicity.

## Harmful effects of drug actions

In another study, ADRs affect around 5%–10% of medical in-patients, and one-half of ADRs occur prior to admission.[2] ADRs can be classified according to dose administered, time course, and susceptibility (DoTS).

Dose can contribute to toxic effects, such as nephrotoxicity with high doses of aminoglycosides; collateral effects, such as *Clostridium difficile* infection with broad-spectrum antibiotics; and hypersusceptibility reactions, which include anaphylactoid reactions to iodinated contrast media and acetylcysteine. ADRs can be time dependent, as in the "red man syndrome," due to rapid administration of vancomycin, or time independent, as seen in ADRs due to drug interactions. Individuals can be vulnerable to ADRs due to genetic variation. Drug can induce hemolysis in patients with glucose-6-phosphate dehydrogenase deficiency. Other factors increasing susceptibility include age, sex, and pathological status of patients. Detecting and reporting ADRs make treatment strategy safer and more likely to achieve its aims especially in combination therapy.

Older populations are more susceptible to drug toxicity in terms of pharmacokinetics and degree of vulnerability to ADRs. Frail older people or those with multiple morbidities often suffer from the adverse drug toxicity, which remains a challenge in caring for older people, as drug doses may not be compromised to reduce risks of ADRs.[3] The majority of ADRs in older people can be avoided by prescribed medications in combination with herbal medicine or phytochemical compounds. The reduction of ADRs is therefore a clinical priority. There is good evidence for ADRs as part of a multifactorial intervention to reduce health risk in health care of the elderly. Multiple medications also contribute to ADRs resulting in mortality particularly in frail older people. *C. difficile* was reported to be associated with use of antibiotics, which mainly affects frail older people leading to substantial morbidity and mortality. Antipsychotics were also reported to increase the risk of stroke by more than threefold in patients with dementia. However, close monitoring and regular medication review of patients can help reduce drug reactions. Use of herbal medicine coupled with prescribed medications would reduce drug toxicity. Individualized medications are helpful to prevent ADRs.

## Management of adverse effects of drug treatment

The management of adverse effects of androgen-deprivation therapy (ADT) can be difficult due to complications related to drug treatment. All relevant medical literature on men with prostate cancer treated with ADT from 2005 to 2014, and older relevant papers reported that there were undesirable adverse effects of ADT that require pro-active prevention and treatment.[4] The harmful effects of ADT included cardiovascular disease, diabetes, osteoporosis, cognitive decline, and sexual dysfunction. The study suggested a systematic monitoring and assessment of the harmful effects were necessary in order to prevent or minimize the numerous harmful effects from ADT.

## Liraglutide, an agonist for treatment of diabetes

The glucagon-like peptide-1 (GLP-1) receptor agonist, liraglutide, is a widely used drug for the treatment of type 2 diabetes. Liraglutide is one of several incretin-based agents that are believed to be associated with pancreatitis and pancreas cancer.[5-6] Annona species (Annonaceae) have long been used as traditional herbal medicines by native peoples in tropical areas. Annonaceae extract was used against a variety of illnesses including infectious diseases, cancer, diabetes, and mental disorders.[5] The experimental results from the pharmacological research enable the validation of their health benefits in treatment of diseases. However, more toxicity assays and clinical trials would be necessary to establish safe doses of prescribed drug and herbal medicine.

## ADRs toward cellular activity

The prevalence and characteristics of ADRs and drug–drug interactions (DDIs) affect treatment of various diseases especially in older adults. A previous study suggested that DDIs significantly contribute to the onset of ADRs in older adults and intervention programmes using big data analysis. A computerized system analysis may reduce the burden of iatrogenic illnesses in the elderly.[7] Brusatol, a natural quassinoid isolated from Traditional Chinese Medicine (TCM) known as Fructus Bruceae, has recently been reported to be an anticancer compound. Fructus Bruceae displayed powerful cytotoxic effects against various types of cell lines including cancer cells. However, the molecular mechanism of actions of Fructus Bruceae remains poorly understood in hepatocellular carcinoma (HCC). A previous study demonstrated that brusatol inhibited cell viability, proliferation, and induced apoptosis in liver cancer lines through inhibition of The phosphatidylinositol 3-kinase (PI3K)/a serine/threonine kinase (Akt)/mammalian target of rapamycin (mTOR) pathways. The PI3K/Akt/mTOR pathway regulates several normal cellular functions that are also critical for tumorigenesis, including cellular proliferation, growth, survival and mobility. The results revealed that brusatol effectively inhibited proliferation and induced apoptosis in HCC through autophagy induction and inhibited tumor invasion and migration *in vivo* and *in vitro*. The findings suggested that brusatol is an anti-tumor agent or a supplement to the current chemotherapeutic systematic plan.[8]

# Benefits of TCM formulations in medical strategy

Fuzi is the processed lateral roots of *Aconitum carmichaelii* Debx (Ranunculaceae), which is a traditional herbal medicine well known for its pharmacological effects and acute toxicity. Aconitum alkaloids are responsible for its pharmacological activity and toxicity. Although a large number of studies on Fuzi have been reported, no comprehensive review on its pharmacokinetics has yet been published.

The use of Fuzi as a personalized medicine based on the bioavailability barrier (BB), which mainly comprises drug-metabolizing enzymes (DMEs) and efflux transporters (ETs), was reported.[9] The study showed that the *Aconitum* alkaloids were rapidly absorbed in the intestine and extensively distributed in the body. DMEs, especially CYP3A4/5, are responsible for various types of metabolic reactions of the *Aconitum* alkaloids. ETs, including P-glycoprotein (P-gp), multidrug resistance-associated protein 2 (MRP2), and breast cancer resistance protein (BCRP), were involved in the efflux of the diester-diterpene alkaloids (DDAs) and name of alkaloid drugs (MDAs). The results indicated kidney toxicity was associated with DDAs in Fuzi. However, the exact toxicological mechanism remains sketchy. The significant impact of Fuzi on DMEs and ETs suggests that the co-administration of Fuzi with drugs that are substrates of DMEs and/or ETs may cause herb–drug interactions (HDIs).[9] Polymorphisms of DMEs and specific drug transporters contribute to the differences in the efficacy and toxicity of Fuzi among individuals. In the future, the use of TCM formulations as personalized medicine is necessary as a complementary treatment strategy in order to achieve therapeutic efficacy with reduced toxicity of drugs.

# Effects of antibiotics and ADRs

Adverse reactions are recognized hazards in health care. A study revealed that the incidence is more in case of antibiotics and ADRs to antibiotics are common and some of them resulted in increased healthcare cost due to the need of some interventions and increased length of hospital stay.[10] In spite of advances in antibiotics, urinary tract infection (UTI) is still among the most common reasons for antibiotic medication. *Persicaria capitata* (Buch.-Ham. ex D. Don) H. Gross (*P. capitata*) is a herbal medicine used in China to treat UTI. However, its mechanism remain unclear. Relinqing® granule, which is made from aqueous extracts of the whole *P. capitata* plant, showed that after the treatments of mice, urine levels of itaconic acid in Relinqing® group increased by 4.9-fold and 11.3-fold compared with model and ciprofloxacin groups, respectively. Itaconic acid is an endogenous antibacterial metabolite produced by macrophages, which serves as a checkpoint for metabolic fate of macrophage. The findings suggested that herbal medicine can be used to cure UTI through modulation of immune system.[11]

ADRs can cause morbidity and mortality. They occur frequently in patients with severe illness and cancer. It is recognized that pharmacogenetic factors are important in determining susceptibility to ADRs.[12]

## Prevention of undesirable drug reactions

Determination of the outcomes of adverse drug events (ADEs) in cancer patients is useful in order to introduce medical intervention related to a drug toxicity. It was reported that 57 ADEs (64.8%) were life threatening, 30 (34.1%) were significant, 1 (1.1%) was fatal, and 14 (15.9%) of all ADEs were preventable.[13] The most common drug classes associated with ADEs were antidiabetics, antibiotics, and analgesics. Critically ill patients with cancer are at high risk of developing ADEs. Treatment strategies that can reduce the incidence and severity of ADEs are essential to improve the treatment efficacy of cancer patients. An alternative approach to cancer therapy with western cancer drug in combination with herbal medicine or anticancer phytochemical compounds becomes a useful complementary strategy in treatment options.

Cancer can be a terminal disease affecting thousands of people every year. Multiple factors such as epigenetics and dietary factors are responsible for abnormal cell growth and cancer. Breast cancer is the most common malignancy among women worldwide, but the long-term hormone therapy is frequently associated with adverse side effects. Tamoxifen is the most widely used specific drug anti-estrogen for the treatment of hormone-dependent breast cancer. However, tamoxifen is effective for cancer patients with estrogen receptor-positive breast cancer. Tamoxifen reduces the risk of recurrence and mortality from breast cancer when given as adjuvant therapy with TCM and provides effective palliation for patients with metastatic breast cancer.[14]

# Use of herbal formula in ameliorating drug toxicity

Danzhi Xiaoyao powder (DXP) is a herbal formula that has an effect on breast cancer, especially estrogen or progesterone, hormone-receptor positive (ER)-positive breast cancer.[15] However, the active compounds and the molecular mechanism of its action against cancer remain unclear. It was reported that a network pharmacology approach comprising drug metabolism, molecular targets, and breast cancer gene collection was useful in cancer therapy. The results suggested that ER-positive breast cancer network, compound–compound target network of DXP, DXP-ER-positive breast cancer network, and compound-known target-ER-positive breast cancer network were helpful in setting up treatment strategy with herbal medicine. Some ER-positive breast cancer and DXP-related targets, clusters, biological processes, and pathways, and several potential anticancer compounds were found. The network analysis successfully predicted the molecular synergy of DXP for ER-positive breast cancer and potential anticancer active compounds and the potential ER-positive breast cancer-associated targets and the related pathways.[14–15] The study provides insights into exploring ethnopharmacological of herbal medicine and multidrug interaction. The treatment strategy with herbal medicine offers exciting prospects that lie ahead.

## Bisphosphonate use in cancer therapy

An adverse event resulting from bisphosphonate (BP) use in cancer therapy was reported. BP-induced renal injury and abnormal cell growth was shown. Effectiveness of zoledronic acid (ZOL) ($n = 411$, 87.5%) and pamidronate ($n = 8$, 17%), and alendronate ($n = 36$, 2%) was recorded.[16] Outcomes reflected a nonsignificant safety signal for the drugs. Acute kidney injury was identified in BP-induced cancer. It was considered that acute kidney injury is attributed to an ADR of BPs and could lead to cancer.[16]

## Effects of chloroquine, an autophagy inhibitor in cancer therapy

Cancer cells deplete energy in tissues through autophagy in metastatic environment. A number of clinical trials revealed the promising role of chloroquine, an autophagy inhibitor, as a novel antitumor drug in cancer therapy.[17]

However, the kidneys are vulnerable to chemotherapeutic agents. Recent studies have shown that TCM plays a protective role against acute kidney injury.[13–17] Cancer drugs such as cisplatin induced kidney injury. It is believed that the use of chloroquine in combination with anticancer drugs may exacerbate kidney damage. Moreover, organs including kidney and liver in which autophagy plays a homeostatic role may be sensitive to the combined use of chloroquine and anticancer drugs. Thus, the use of TCM in cancer and kidney injury, especially on the use of chloroquine to treat cancer, can be beneficial. The possible side effects in the combined use of chloroquine and anticancer drugs would be reduced.

## Undesirable drug reactions in children

ADRs in children are of major concern nowadays. A systematic review of observational studies in children showed that ADRs might be better detected, assessed, and avoided. [18]The study indicated the primary outcome was clinical event described as an ADR to one or more drugs. Incidence rates for ADRs causing hospital admission ranged from 0.4% to 10.3% of all children tested (estimate of 2.9%) and from 0.6% to 16.8% of all children exposed to a drug during hospital stay. Anti-infective agents and anti-epileptics were the most frequently reported cases associated with ADRs in children admitted to hospital, while anti-infective agents and nonsteroidal anti-inflammatory drugs (NSAIDs) were frequently reported as associated with ADRs in outpatient children. However, ADRs can be avoidable or reduced. Nevertheless, further work is needed to address how ADRs may be prevented.

Although ADRs and DDIs frequently happen, few studies have looked at the epidemiology of ADEs in oncology. It is helpful to investigate how cancer drugs are related to a DDI or an ADR. A previous study showed from September 2007 to May 2008 in a hospital, 39 patients (13.0%, 95% confidence interval [CI] 9.4%–17.4%) were considered to be associated with an ADE, 33 (11.0%, 95% CI 7.7%–15.2%) with an ADR, and 6 (2.0%, 95% CI 0.7%–4.3%) with a DDI.[19] One of the most common DDIs involved warfarin, captopril, and anti-inflammatory agents, and the most frequent ADR was neutropenic fever post-chemotherapy. Approximately 1 in 10 cancer patients is associated with an ADE. Prospective and population-based studies are warranted to evaluate their magnitude in oncology and the use of TCM to reduce incidence of DDI and ADRs.

## Drug toxicity of doxorubicin

One of the common drugs for treatment of different types of cancer is doxorubicin, which is an anthracyline drug first extracted from *Streptomyces peucetius* var. *caesius* in the 1970s and routinely used in the treatment of cancer including breast, lung, gastric, ovarian, thyroid, non-Hodgkin's and Hodgkin's lymphoma, multiple myeloma, sarcoma, and pediatric cancers.[20] A major limitation for the use of doxorubicin is cardiotoxicity. The study showed that the mechanism of anticancer actions and of cardiotoxicity occurs through different pathways. It is hoped that analogous compounds with equal efficacy can be developed but with reduced toxicity. However, the pharmacogenomics of these pathways remains unclear. Nevertheless, the candidate genes for the pharmacogenomics of doxorubicin action in a stylized cancer cell and toxicity in cardiomyocytes were reported.[20]

## Prediction of adverse side reactions of novel compounds

A common feature of cancer patients is loss of lean tissue, specifically skeletal muscle, which may be associated with side effects of chemotherapy or drugs especially with high dose of drugs. It was reported that lean tissue loss has adverse implications for toxicity of antineoplastic therapy and cancer prognosis.[21] Contemporary cancer populations have been shown to have heterogeneous proportions of lean tissue, regardless of body weight. Wasting of lean tissue has triggered tumor progression and reduced survival. Lean tissue depletion is a reliable predictor of severe drug toxicity in patients treated with chemotherapeutic agents. Muscle loss can be attributed to side effects of a chemotherapeutic agent including sorafenib, statins, and androgen suppression therapy. However, the risk of an ADR can vary considerably among patients, and the epigenetic and dietary factors including medical supplements with TCM can ameliorate an individual's susceptibility to an adverse reaction. The treatment strategy may include genetically determined alterations in drug response and concurrent pathological conditions of patients.[22]

ADRs represent one of the main health and economic problems in the world. With increasing data on ADRs, there is an increased need for alternative medicine with TCM and/or phytochemicals for the treatment strategy. In addition, more versatile software tools capable of storing and analysis of the information on drug toxicity and ADR associations would be necessary to enhance drug efficacy. A recent study showed the usefulness of a computational procedure capable of extracting drug-ADR statistical data from the large collection of patient safety reports, which was stored in the Federal Drug Administration database.[23] The study was capable of generating population-specific drug-ADR frequencies and can be made specific to a single patient population group (such as gender or age) or a single therapy characteristic including drug dosage and duration of therapy. However, computational prediction of serious and rare ADRs remains a challenge. Nevertheless current state-of-the-art computational methods yield more reliable predictions of ADRs based on the theory of "compressed sensing" (CS), which can accurately predict side effects of new and established drugs.[24] The method was reported to be able to infer chemical-ADR associations using incomplete databases with accuracy. The results suggested that the prediction accuracy of ADR of new drugs could be increased accordingly.

Small molecules may be used as research tools to probe drug interaction and its mechanistic actions in cells and lead to the development of new therapeutic agents. Some can inhibit a specific function of enzymes in signaling pathways or disrupt drug–protein interactions. Some of the common phytochemicals from herbal medicine are reported in Appendix IV. Small natural molecules readily bind specific biological macromolecules and acts as an effector that can modulate the cellular activity or function of the target, especially cancer cell growth. Small molecules can exhibit a variety of biological functions or applications, serving many other roles in the signaling processes. These phytochemical compounds including secondary metabolites are natural. Some of these phytochemical compounds display a beneficial effect against a disease or may be cytotoxic such as cancer drug candidate.

# References

1. Nagayama, T. (2015). Adverse drug reactions for medicine newly approved in Japan from 1999 to 2013: syncope/loss of consciousness and seizures/convulsions. *Regul Toxicol Pharmacol.*72(3): 572–7. doi: 10.1016/j.yrtph.2015.05.030.

2. Ferner, R.E., and Butt, T.F. (2012). Adverse drug reactions. *Medicine.* 30(7): 366–370 doi:10.1016/j.mpmed.2012.05.001.

3. Davies, E.A., and O'Mahony, M.S. (2015). Adverse drug reactions in special populations - the elderly. *Br J Clin Pharmacol.* 24: 111–125. doi: 10.1111/bcp.12596.

4. Rhee, H., Gunter, J.H., Heathcote, P., *et al.* (2015). Management of cancer drug reactions and diabetes. *BJU Int.* 115(Suppl 5): 3–13. doi: 10.1111/bju.12964.

5. Chalmer, T., Almdal, T.P., Vilsbøll, T., and Knop, F.K. (2015). Adverse drug reactions associated with the use of liraglutide in patients with type 2 diabetes–focus on pancreatitis and pancreas cancer. *Expert Opin Drug Saf.* 14(1): 171–80. doi: 10.1517/14740338.2015.975205.

6. Quilez, A.M., Fernandez-Arche, M.A., and Garcia-Gimenez, M.D. (2018). Potential therapeutic applications of the genus *Annona*: local and traditional uses and pharmacology. *J Ethnopharmacol.* 225: 244–270.

7. Marengoni, A., Pasina, L., Concoreggi, C., *et al.* (2014). Understanding adverse drug reactions in older adults through drug-drug interactions. *Eur J Intern Med.* 25(9): 843–846. doi: 10.1016/j.ejim.2014.10.001.

8. Ruifan, Y., Ninggao D., and Qikuan H. (2018). Comprehensive anti-tumor effect of brusatol through inhibition of cell viability and promotion of apoptosis caused by autophagy via the PI3K/Akt/mTOR pathway in hepatocellular carcinoma. *Biomed Pharmacother.* 105: 962–973.

9. Wu, J.J., Guo, Z.Z., Zhu, Y.F., *et al.* (2018). A systematic review of pharmacokinetic studies on herbal drug Fuzi: implications for Fuzi as personalized medicine. *Phytomedicine.* 44: 187–203. doi: 10.1016/j.phymed.2018.03.001.

10. Shamna, M., Dilip, C., Ajmal, M., *et al.* (2014). A prospective study on adverse drug reactions of antibiotics in a tertiary care hospital. *Saudi Pharm J.* 22(4): 303–308. doi: 10.1016/j.jsps.2013.06.004.

11. Han, P., Huang, Y., and Xie, Y., (2018).Metabolomics reveals immunomodulation as a possible mechanism for the antibiotic effect of *Persicaria capitata* (Buch.-Ham. ex D. Don). *Metabolomics.* 14 (7): 200–208. Article Number: 91.

12. Scott, S., and Thompson, J. (2014). Adverse drug reactions. *Anaesth Intensive Care Med.* 15(5): 245–249.

13. Nazer, L.H., Hawari, F., and Al-Najjar, T. (2014). Adverse drug events in critically ill patients with cancer: incidence, characteristics, and outcomes. *J Pharm Pract.* 27(2): 208–213. doi: 10.1177/0897190013513302.

14. Yang, G., Nowsheen, S., Aziz, K., and Georgakilas, A.G. (2013). Toxicity and adverse effects of Tamoxifen and other anti-estrogen drugs. *Pharmacol Ther.* 139(3): 392–404. doi: 10.1016/j.pharmthera.2013.05.005.

15. Yang, K., Zeng, L., and Ge, J. (2018). Exploring the pharmacological mechanism of Danzhi Xiaoyao powder on ER-Positive breast cancer by a network pharmacology approach. *Evid Based Complement Altern Med.* 2018(5):101–109. doi: 10.1155/2018/5059743.

16. Edwards, B.J., Usmani, S., Raisch, D.W., *et al.* (2013). Acute kidney injury and bisphosphonate use in cancer: a report from the research on adverse drug events and reports (RADAR). *J Oncol Pract.* 9(2): 101–106. doi: 10.1200/JOP.2011.000486.

17. Kimura, T., Takabatake, Y., Takahashi, A., and Isaka,Y. (2013). Chloroquine in cancer therapy: a double-edged sword of autophagy. *Cancer Res.* 73(1): 3–7. doi: 10.1158/0008-5472.CAN-12-2464.

18. Smyth, R.M., Gargon, E., Kirkham, J., *et al.* (2012). Adverse drug reactions in children– a systematic review. *PLoS ONE.* 7(3): e24061. doi: 10.1371/journal.pone.0024061.

19. Miranda, V., Fede, A., Nobuo, M., *et al.* (2010). Adverse drug reactions and drug interactions as causes of hospital admission in oncology. *J Pain Symptom Manage.* 42(3): 342–353. doi: 10.1016/j.jpainsymman.2010.11.014.

20. Thorn, C.F., Oshiro, C., Marsh, S., *et al.* (2011). Doxorubicin pathways: pharmacodynamics and adverse effects. *Pharmacogenet Genomics.* 21(7): 440–446. doi: 10.1097/FPC.0b013e32833ffb56.

21. Prado, M., Antoun, S., Sawyer, M.B., and Baracos, V.E. (2011). Two faces of drug therapy in cancer: drug-related lean tissue loss and its adverse consequences to survival and toxicity. *Curr Opin Clin Nutr Metab Care.* 14(3): 250–254. doi: 10.1097/MCO.0b013e3283455d45.

22. Ferner, R.E. (2011). What's new in…: Adverse drug reactions. *Medicine.* 39(4): 239–241 doi:10.1016/j.mpmed.2010.12.015.

23. Poleksic, A., Turner, C., Dalal, R., Gray, P., and Xie, L. (2017). Mining FDA resources to compute population-specific frequencies of adverse drug reactions. *Proceedings (IEEE Int Conf Bioinformatics Biomed).* 2017: 1809–1814. doi: 10.1109/BIBM.2017.8217935. Epub 2017 Dec 18

24. Poleksic, A., and Xie, L. (2018). Predicting serious rare adverse reactions of novel chemicals. *Bioinformatics.* 34(16): 2835–2842. doi: 10.1093/bioinformatics/bty193.

# TREATMENT OF CANCER WITH NATURAL PRODUCTS

Cancer incidence and mortality are increasing worldwide. Regardless of advancement of science and technology, cancer therapy remains a challenge due to drug toxicity and drug resistance. The economic impact of current cancer therapy mandates a closer look at alternative and complementary ways to overcome this financial burden of cancer patients. Epidemiological evidence for the association between cancer and epigenetic and dietary factors has prompted the exploration of herbal medicine including natural chemicals from different naturally occurring substances in natural environment. However, drug interactions and the potential toxicity of novel compounds present an obstacle in drug development.

A previous study reported on the use of several whole natural plant extracts and isolated constituents for intervention in an attempt to highlight beneficial effects of natural compounds.[1] Yet the detail of standardized formulation of herbal medicine and systematic assessment of clinical trial of herbal medicine is lacking.

The lack of parallel comparison studies between the extracts and their isolated compounds limits the common use of the treatment strategy with natural products and herbal medicine. It was suggested that a rigorous comparative study of potential anticancer agents and established drugs was helpful in order to identify which one of the natural products would be better qualified to take on the mantle of cancer management.

Drug resistance is a major problem in cancer chemotherapy and was responsible for treatment failure in 90% of patients with metastatic cancer. From the research work in the past 30 years, multi-mechanisms responsible for the development of drug resistance have been identified.[2] However, it remains a challenge to identify single agents that can target specific mechanism of drug resistance. Traditionally, herbs have the potential to target multi-mechanism of drug resistance, cancer, and malignant neoplasm since herbal extracts contain multiple components that may act on multiple molecular targets and related signaling processes. An early study provided an overview of the known mechanisms of drug resistance and useful information on herbal medicines as therapeutic agents.[2] It was found that some of the medicinal herbs are capable of inducing strong anticancer effect with various mechanisms, but relevant information useful for development of herbs as viable products for therapeutic use is generally inadequate. Ideas for improving *in vitro* and *in vivo* screening tests prior to clinical studies could help development of herbal product as anticancer agent for the treatment of various types of cancer.

## Overcome multidrug resistance with natural products

Overexpression of P-glycoprotein (P-gp) and multidrug resistance-associate protein 1 (MRP1) is a major mechanism leading to multidrug resistance (MDR) of cancer cells. These transporters expel anticancer drugs and greatly impair therapeutic efficacy of chemotherapy.[3] A Chinese herbal plant Yanhusuo (*Corydalis yanhusuo*) is frequently used in functional food and TCM to improve the efficacy of chemotherapy. Effects of glaucine, an alkaloid component of Yanhusuo, on P-gp and MRP1 in resistant cancer cells were reported. The resistant cancer cell line, MCF-7/ADR, and corresponding parental sensitive cells were employed to determine reversal properties of glaucine. Glaucine was shown to inhibit P-gp and MRP1-mediated efflux and activate ATPase activities of the transporters, indicating that it was a substrate and inhibited P-gp and MRP1 competitively. Also glaucine displayed inhibition of expression of ABC transporter genes. It reverses the resistance of MCF-7/ADR to adriamycin (ADM) and mitoxantrone effectively. However, the active ingredients of Yanhusuo extract remained unclear.

Another study reported the therapeutic effects of stephania tetrandra-containing Chinese herbal formula on reversing MDR of chemotherapy in lung cancer cell line, SW1573/2R120.[4] It was shown that chemotherapeutic drug resistance in lung cancer was mainly due to high expression of MRP gene and activation of caspases. The effect of *Stephania tetrandra*-containing Chinese herbal formula, namely Supplement Energy and Nourish Lung (SENL), is effective in enhancing efficacy and reducing toxicity of chemotherapy in lung cancer. However, the underlying mechanism is largely unknown. Nevertheless, the study suggested how SENL herbs function on multidrug-resistance lung cancer cells. The effects of SENL herbs alone or together with a chemotherapeutic drug, ADM, were assessed. The results showed that SENL herbs had a significant synergistic effect with ADM in inhibiting the growth of SW 1573/2R120 cells. Either SENL alone or together with ADM could significantly increase cell apoptosis via mitochondria- and caspase-dependent pathway. Furthermore, SENL herbs were able to reverse drug resistance of lung cancer cell line by decreasing MRP expression and increasing accumulation of intracellular ADM. Taken together, the results suggested that the mechanistic actions of SENL underlying reversal effect of drug resistance were through apoptotic activity and caspase cascade. The study sheds light on the mechanism of drug resistance and how to enhance efficacy of cancer therapy.

Persistent cancer chemotherapy can induce MDR, which is one of the major reasons for failure of chemotherapy. The ABCB1 transporter is a member of the ATP-binding cassette superfamily, and it is frequently over-expressed in multidrug resistant cancer cells. Active ingredients derived from TCM have been reported to reverse MDR mediated by ATP-binding cassette transporters. A study showed that acerinol, isolated from *Cimicifuga acerina*, was tested for its effects on the ABCB1 transporter. The results demonstrated that acerinol could increase the chemosensitivity of ABCB1-overexpressing HepG2/ADM and MCF-7/ADR cells to chemotherapeutic drugs, doxorubicin (DOX), vincristine, and paclitaxel. [5] Furthermore, it could increase the retention of ABCB1 substrates DOX and rhodamine 123 in HepG2/ADM and MCF-7/ADR cells. The results indicated that acerinol significantly stimulated the activity of ABCB1 ATPase without affecting the gene expression of ABCB1 and was found to be able to reverse the resistance of MCF-7/ADR cells to vincristine. The reversibility of acerinol action suggested that acerinol may act as a competitive inhibitor of ABCB1 by competing with drugs as substrates such as DOX. Docking analysis indicated that acerinol would bind to the active sites on ABCB1 overlapping with that of verapamil. Taken together, acerinol could significantly enhance the cytotoxicity of chemotherapeutic drugs by modulating the actions of ABCB1 in cancer cells. Acerinol shows promise as a new MDR reversal agent.

## Beta-elemene, an inhibitor of P-gp activity

Other study indicated that beta-elemene, a compound isolated from the Chinese herbal medicine *Curcuma wenyujin*, was capable of reversing tumor MDR although the mechanism remains elusive.[6] The study showed beta-elemene treatment markedly increased accumulation of DOX and rhodamine 123 in both K562/DNR and SGC7901/ADR cells and significantly inhibited the expression of P-gp. Beta-elemene significantly induced downregulation of Akt phosphorylation and upregulation of the E3 ubiquitin ligases, c-Cbl and Cbl-b. Also, beta-elemene was shown to significantly enhance the antitumor activity of DOX in nude mice bearing SGC7901/ADR xenografts. The study suggested that beta-elemene might target P-gp overexpressing leukemia and cancer cells to enhance the efficacy of DOX. Taken together, the results were correlated with the previous study in which overexpression of P-gp and MRP1 was associated with MDR in cancer cells.[3]

## Tanshinone I inhibits P-gp activity

Tanshinones are diterpene quinones. They are isolated from *Salvia miltiorrhiza* Bunge (Lamiaceae), which is also known as "Danshen." Danshen extracts have been studied for anticancer potential in various cancer cell lines *in vitro* and in tumor-bearing mice. Four structurally similar tanshinones including dihydrotanshinone, tanshinone I, tanshinone IIA, and cryptotanshinone were identified and shown to exhibit anticancer activities through caspase cascade in a hepatoma cell line (HepG2)[7] and metastatic melanoma cell lines.[8] Among these four diterpene quinones, dihydrotanshinone showed higher cytotoxicity in P-gp-overexpressing DOX-resistant HepG2 (R-HepG2) than other three tanshinones tested.[9,10] The findings indicated that dihydrotanshinone induced apoptosis through p38 mitogen-activated protein kinase (MAPK) phosphorylation.[11]

The bio-availability of tanshinone IIA and tanshinone IIB is limited by the presence of P-gp although both compounds are P-gp substrates. However, only tanshinone I inhibited P-gp.[12] The results suggest the bio-availability of tanshinones determined the beneficial effects of tanshinones *in vivo* study.

# Natural polyphenols in cancer therapy

Natural polyphenols are the major class of phytochemical compounds present in plants, which are characterized by the presence of phenolic functionality.[13] The molecular weight of natural polyphenols ranges from 500 to 4000 Da arranged in five to seven aromatic rings per 1000 Da.[14] However, only polyphenols with lower molecular weight have been shown to have potential benefits in humans or anticancer activity.[15]

Four main classes of polyphenols have been classified as follows[16]:

**(A)** Phenolic acids
**(B)** Flavonoids
**(C)** Stilbenes
**(D)** Lignans

The implications of polyphenols in human health include beneficial effects in cancer therapy,[17] neuroprotection,[18] cardiovascular system dysfunction and damage,[19] the metabolic syndrome,[20] diabetes,[21] and different inflammation-related pathologies.[22] It was reported that polyphenols could modulate cellular longevity through histone posttranslational modification and induce the upregulation of autophagy, thus reducing the level of acetyl coenzyme A (AcCoA). In addition, the effect of caloric restriction (CR) on cancer-related chronic inflammation was ameliorated in aging.[22] Consequently, SIRT1 protein levels were increased in response to calorie restriction mimetics (CRM) and acted as autophagy inducers to cancer therapy.[23,24] Polyphenols have been used for thousands of years in folk medicine. Although *in vitro* studies of polyphenols show promise, the *in vivo* experiments indicate poor correlations with the *in vitro* results. Incorporation of these compounds into western medicine for treatment of diseases remains to be further exploited.

Natural polyphenols are secondary metabolites of plants that play an important role in the defense against carnivores, pathogens, and other organisms. Some of these active natural polyphenols are shown to exhibit health benefits.[17]

The following four natural polyphenols are shown to exhibit strong anticancer activities:

**(1)** (−)-Epigallocatechin-3-gallate (EGCG) is abundant in green tea
**(2)** Curcumin is a major component of turmeric,

(3)  Resveratrol, a phytoalexin found in grapes, red wine, and mulber-
ries

(4)  Pterostilbene, a natural resveratrol analogue.

These active polyphenols have been shown in the treatment of cancer.

*In vitro* studies show that EGCG, curcumin, or resveratrol sensitizes
cancer cell line (LNCaP) prostate cancer cells to TNF-related apoptosis
inducing ligand (TRAIL)-mediated apoptosis through modulation of the
extrinsic apoptotic pathway.[25,26] Moreover, EGCG inhibited cell growth
and induced apoptosis by inhibition of Fas in cells with high levels of Fas
activity such as LNCaP. EGCG was also shown to inhibit fatty acid synthase
in intact cells and selectively induce apoptosis in prostate cancer cells.[27]
Furthermore, polyphenols can also induce apoptosis by intrinsic pathway
by activating caspases-9 and -3 and by changing the Bax/Bcl-2 ratio,[28] and
similar effects were observed with EGCG,[29] curcumin,[30] or pterostilbene[31]
in different cancer cell lines. Although the *in vitro* and *in vivo* studies of
anticancer properties of some of these natural polyphenols were reported,
the details of bioavailability and apoptotic actions of individual polyphenols remain sketchy.

## Molecular targets of natural polyphenols

Characterization of novel molecular targets of active natural polyphenols
would provide clue for development of specific antitumor agents with reduced
side effects. At present, strategies of cancer treatment using the combination of
targeted therapies and chemotherapies or radiotherapies offer better survival.
However, malignant cells may develop drug resistance. Indeed, changing conditions within tissue microenvironments and weakened immune system can
cause alterations in the metastatic cells leading to cancer growth.

Most of the natural polyphenols are known to exhibit inhibitory effects
on different types of cancer and signaling processes. It was reported that tea
polyphenols and atorvastatin synergistically inhibited murine lung tumorigenesis and the growth of lung cancer H1299 and H460 cells through
caspase cascade.[32] Another study showed that epicatechin enhanced the
induction of growth inhibition and apoptosis in human lung cancer cells
by curcumin.[33]

Although there is a large number of polyphenols that have been
identified with medicinal properties, a limited number of active natural

polyphenols exhibit strong anticancer activities. Nevertheless, the anti-cancer activities of active polyphenols vary among different types of cancer. The differences in chemical structure and molecular size of natural polyphenols present limitations to the bioactivity and bioavailability of the active polyphenols *in vivo* study.

# Resveratrol

It was first detected in dried roots of *Polygonum cuspidatum*. It is a member of the stilbene family and can be found in isoforms *cis-* and *trans-*, being *trans*-resveratrol is the more abundant natural isoform.[34] The ability of resveratrol to induce carcinogenic inhibition was reported in 1997.[35] Resveratrol was found to act as an antioxidant and antimutagen and to induce phase II drug-metabolizing enzymes. It was reported that *trans*-resveratrol was able to mediate anti-inflammatory effects and inhibited cyclooxygenase and hydroperoxidase functions and induced differentiation of human promyelocytic leukemia cell. Although the antitumor effects of resveratrol have been reported, detail of its mechanism of action in cancer cells remains unclear. Numerous studies showed that resveratrol could induce apoptosis via p53 activation, modulate cell cycle alterations, caspase activity induction,[36–38] downregulation of Bcl-2, Bcl-xL, survivin levels, and upregulation of Bax levels,[39] Bak, PUMA, Noxa, Bim, TRAIL-R1/DR4, and TRAIL-R2/DR5.[40]

Phosphorylation of P53 prevented the binding with Mouse double minute 2 homolog (MDM2)[41] and facilitated the acetylation of P53 at a C-terminal lysine.[42] P53 acetylation increased sequence-specific DNA binding and subsequently disrupted the DNA activity. Moreover, it was shown that treatment of a mutant P53 prostate cancer DU145 cells with resveratrol-induced phosphorylation of Ser-15, which restored wild-type P53 DNA binding and P53 acetylation,[43] activating pro-apoptotic events. In addition, resveratrol was also shown to phosphorylate Ser-15 and induce expression of various P53-regulated p21, Bax, Fas, caspase 8/9 activation, and decrease Bcl-2 expression in in MCF7 breast carcinoma cells.[44]

It was reported that resveratrol also inhibited the IKB kinase complex (IKK)-mediated IβB phosphorylation by stimulating the retention of nuclear factor (NF)-kappa B (NFκB) in the cytosol and its subsequent inactivation of signaling process would lead to apoptosis.[45] The results indicated that resveratrol inhibited cell proliferation and caused cell cycle arrest.[46]

## Curcumin, a phenolic compound derived from medicinal plants

Curcumin, a phenolic compound derived from rhizome of the plant *Curcuma longa*, was known to exhibit anti-inflammatory and anticancer activity.[47] Nowadays, curcumin is recognized by the US Food and Drug Administration as generally recognized as safe (GRAS) phytochemicals. *In vitro* and *in vivo* experiments have shown that curcumin could sensitize tumor cells to TRAIL-induced apoptosis, inhibit NFκB activity, and downregulate expression of the antiapoptotic Bcl-2, Bcl-xL, and XIAP proteins.[48] Moreover, curcumin was shown to upregulate expression of P53, Bax, Bak, PUMA, Bim, NOXA, and death receptors DR4 and DR5, triggering activation of caspase-3, -9, -7, and inducing polyadenosine 5'diphosphateribosediphosphateribose polymerase (PARP) in myeloma cell lines.[49]

An early study also demonstrated that curcumin modulated gene expression in glioblastoma U251 cells and increased cellular levels of DAPk1.[50]

Moreover, curcumin inhibited the activity of signal transducer and activator of transcription 3 (STAT3), a transcription factor that plays an important function in cell growth and apoptosis regulation in glioma cells. However, the exact mechanisms underlying DAPk1 regulation by curcumin, pro-apoptotic effects of curcumin, and regulation of STAT3 and NF-κB pathways and caspase-3 inhibition remain unclear.

## Pterostilbene

Pterostilbene (*trans*-3,5-dimethoxy-4-hydroxystilbene) is a natural resveratrol analogue but significantly more bioavailable in plasma when ingested.[51] Although their pharmacological properties are very similar, pterostilbene exhibited higher lipophilic properties that facilitated its cellular uptake. The difference in chemical structure of resveratrol and its analogue contributes to the differences in bioactivity and bioavailability of stilbene in animal study.

Pterostilbene was shown to induce mitochondrial membrane depolarization with a subsequent activation of the caspase cascade in various cancer cell lines including breast (MCF7),[52] bladder (T24),[53] colon (HT29),[54] myeloid leukemia cells (HL-60, K562),[55] and lung cancer cell lines including A549, H460, and SK-MES-1 and pancreatic cancer (MIA PaCa, PANC-1),[56] prostate (PC3),[52] and human gastric carcinoma cells.[57] Although the results showed the anticancer effects of resveratrol through activation of the intrinsic pathway, the apoptotic mechanisms induced by pterostilbene are not completely understood in different cancer cell lines. Other studies demonstrated the ability of pterostilbene to inhibit cell growth by inducing cell cycle arrest and to alter expression of cell cycle regulators such as P53 and retinoblastoma protein.[36] The results showed that pterostilbene promoted cancer cell death via a mechanism involving lysosomal membrane permeabilization depending on their lysosomal heat shock protein 70 (HSP70) content, which is a known stabilizer of lysosomal membranes.[36,58]

It was reported that oncogenic activation of the KRAS gene via point mutations occurred in 20%–30% of patients with nonsmall cell lung cancer (NSCLC).[59] The RAS-RAF-ERK and RAS-PI3-KAKT pathways were induced downstream in RAS mutation, leading to cancer and their metastasis. A new pharmacological KRAS signaling inhibitor krukovine, which is a small molecular bisbenzylisoquinoline alkaloid, isolated from the bark of *Abuta grandifolia* (Mart.) Sandw. (Menispermaceae), was shown to target the KRAS downstream signaling pathways in different NSCLC cell lines, such as H460 and A549. The study showed the anticancer activities of krukovine in KRAS-mutated NSCLC and other lung cancer cell lines through the induction of cell apoptosis and G1 arrest and by inactivating AKT signaling pathway and downregulating the RAF-ERK signaling pathway.[60,61] Krukovine also suppressed the C-RAF, ERK, AKT, PI3K, p70s6k, and the mechanistic target of rapamycin (mTOR) phosphorylation in H460 and A549.[62,63] The study provides insights into mechanism of anticancer isoquinoline alkaloids in cancer cells. However, the development of KRAS inhibitors including farnesyltransferase inhibitors was reported. Nevertheless, the effectiveness of these inhibitors in cancer cells appeared to be insignificant.[62] Although several AKT inhibitors have been developed and subjected to clinical trials for NSCLC treatment, their adverse side effects, such as severe hyperglycemia and other potential metabolic abnormalities, hinder their applications.

# Natural products as anticancer agents

Since 1961, many medicinal plants provide an excellent source of anticancer agents in the USA. A number of plant- and herb-derived anticancer agents have been approved by FDA including vinca alkaloids, e.g., vinblastine (Vel-ban), vincristine (Oncovin); podophyllotoxins, e.g., etoposide, teniposide; taxoids, e.g., taxol (paclitaxel); navelbine (vinorelbine); taxotere (docetaxel); and cam-potethins, e.g., camptothecin (Camptosar), topotecan (Hycamtin), and irinotecan.[64] Research in herbal compounds has intensified in order to develop novel drugs for treatment of various diseases including cancer. Kaempferol-apigenin, was isolated from the leaves of *Jacaranda acutifolia*,[65] oleanane-type saponins from the leaves of *Albizia anthelmintica* Brongn.[66] Table 10.1 listed some of the common natural polyphenols and their pharmacological activities in cells.

**Table 10.1**  Some common natural polyphenols used as complementary medicine in cancer therapy

| Phytochemicals | Therapeutic activity | Reference |
|---|---|---|
| Curcumin | Protective effects against cancers including gastrointestinal, genitourinary, gynecological, hematological, pulmonary, thymic, brain, breast, and bone | Shehzad et al.[67], Darvesh et al.[68] |
| Tanshinone IIA | To induce gastric cancer cell growth inhibition and apoptosis in a time- and concentration-dependent manner | Chen et al[69] |
| Epigallocatechin gallate (EGCG) | To activate mitogen-activated protein kinase (MAPK) pathway, leading to expression of survival genes<br>Activate caspase pathway and apoptosis | Ali et al.[70], Chung et al.[71] |
| Theaflavin | To inhibit purified 20S proteasome<br>→ Suppression of tumor cell proliferation | Ali et al.[70], Mujtaba et al.[72] |
| Sapogenol | Suppression of cell growth<br>Antiproliferative activity against MCF-7 breast cancer cell | Ali et al.[70], Kinjo et al.[73] |
| Baicalin | To exhibit cytotoxic effect on leukemia-derived T-cells | Ueda et al.[74] |
| Balanitin-6 and balanitin-7 | Anticancer effects against A549 nonsmall-cell lung cancer and U373 glioblastoma cell lines | Ali et al.[70] |

More recent study reported that ethanol herbal extract of *Luffa cylindrica* leaves exhibited anticancer activities on different types of breast cancer cell lines including MCF-7, BT-474, and MDA-MB-231.[75]

Breast cancer is one of the most prevalent cancer worldwide. Development of novel drugs and active phytochemicals is warranted to provide complementary treatment of breast cancer. A recent study suggested the mechanism of anticancer activity of ethanol herbal extract of *L. cylindrica* leaves was through induction of intrinsic and the related signaling pathways leading to inhibition of cell growth. The analysis of the major active constituents of the extract revealed the presence of phenolic compound derivatives and saponin that may be responsible in part for the activity of the extract. However, detail of the chemical properties of the chemical ingredients is lacking.

Natural polyphenols show multi-arrays of biologic and pharmacologic activities, yet their bioavailability in *in vivo* animal models seriously limits their development as therapeutics. A combination of metabolomics-based screening and quality consistency control (MSQCC) of active natural polyphenols and their synthetic analogues may provide a practical approach to this long-standing problem. A recent study showed that the method offered the co-correlation screen of metabolomic and biological profiles of 180 fractions prepared from natural heterogeneous biologic samples as a way to identify a series of bufadinolides as quality control markers for inhibitors of cancer cell.[76] The methodology provides a strategy for large-scale screening test and application of the control markers in quality assurance.

# References

1. Hussain, S.S., Kumar, A.P., and Ghosh, R. (2016). Food-based natural products for cancer management: is the whole greater than the sum of the parts? *Semin Cancer Biol.* 41: 233–246. doi: 10.1016/j.semcancer.2016.06.002.
2. Wang, Z., Chen, X., Huang, Y., Lam, C.W.K., and Chow, M.S.S. (2014). Overcoming chemotherapy resistance with herbal medicines: past, present and future perspectives. *Phytochem Rev.* 13(1): 323–337. doi: 10.1007/s11101-013-9327-z.
3. Lei, Y., Tan, J., Wink, M., Ma, Y.G., Li, N., and Su, G.N. (2012). An isoquinoline alkaloid from the Chinese herbal plant *Corydalis yanhusuo* WT Wang inhibits P-glycoprotein and multidrug resistance-associate protein 1. *Food Chem.* 136(3): 1117–1121. doi: 10.1016/j.foodchem.2012.09.059.
4. Xu, M., Sheng, L.H., Zhu,X.H., Zeng, S.B., and Zhang, G.J. (2010). Reversal effect of *Stephania tetrandra*-containing Chinese herb formula SENL on multidrug resistance in lung cancer cell line SW1573/2R120. *Am J Chinese Med.* 38(2): 401–413. doi. org/10.1142/S0192415X10007919.

5. Liu, D.L., Li, Y.J., Yao, N., *et al.* (2014). Acerinol, a cyclolanstane triterpenoid from *Cimicifuga acerina*, reverses ABCB1-mediated multidrug resistance in HepG2/ADM and MCF-7/ADR cells. *Eur J Pharmacol.* 733: 34–44. doi: 10.1016/j.ejphar.2014.03.043.

6. Zhang, Y., Mu, X.D., Li, E.Z., *et al.* (2013). The role of E3 ubiquitin ligase Cbl proteins in beta-elemene reversing multi-drug resistance of human gastric adenocarcinoma cells. *Int J Mol Sci.* 14 (5): 10075–10089. doi: 10.3390/ijms140510075.

7. Chiu, C.M., Huang, S.Y., Chang, S.F., Liao, K.F., and Chiu, S.C. (2018). Synergistic anti-tumor effects of tanshinone IIA and sorafenib or its derivative SC-1 in hepatocellular carcinoma cells. *Oncotargets Ther.* 11: 1777–1785. doi: 10:2147/OTT.S161534.

8. Saraf, R.S., Datta, A., Sima, C.H., Lopes, R., and Bittner, M. (2018). An in-silico study examining the induction of apoptosis by cryptotanshinone in metastatic melanoma cell lines. *BMC Cancer.* 18: 855–862. doi: 10.1186/s12885-018-4756-0.

9. Hu, T., Wang, L., Zhang, L., *et al.* (2015). Sensitivity of apoptosis-resistant colon cancer cells to tanshinones is mediated by autophagic cell death and p53-independent cyto-toxicity. *Phytomedicine.* 22(5): 536–544. doi: 10.1016/j.phymed.2015.03.010.

10. Hu, T., To, K.K.W., Wang, L., *et al.* (2014). Reversal of P-glycoprotein (P-gp) mediated multidrug resistance in colon cancer cells by cryptotanshinone and dihydrotanshi-none of *Salvia miltiorrhiza*. *Phytomedicine.* 21 (11): 1264–1272. doi.org/10.1016./j.phymed.2014.06.013.

11. Zhou, X., Wang, Y., Lee, W.Y.W.,et al. (2015). Miltirone is a dual inhibitor of P-glycoprotein and cell growth in doxorubicin-resistant HepG2 cells. *J Nat Prod.* 78(9): 2266–2275. doi: 10.1021/acs.jnatprod.5b00516

12. Li, H., and Lai. H. (2017).Tanshinone IIA enhances the chemosensitivity of breast can-cer cells to doxorubicin through down-regulating the expression of MDR-related ABC transporters. *Biomed Pharmacother.* 96: 371–377. doi: 10.1016/j.biopha.2017.10.016

13. Dai, J., and Mumper, R.J. (2010). Plant phenolics: extraction, analysis and their antiox-idant and anticancer properties. *Molecules.* 15: 7313–7352.

14. Quideau, S., Deffieux, D., Douat-Casassus, C., and Pouysegu, L. (2011). Plant polyphenols: chemical properties, biological activities, and synthesis. *Angew Chem Int Ed. Engl.* 50(3): 586–621.

15. Sies, H. (2010). Polyphenols and health: update and perspectives. *Arch Biochem Bio-phys.* 501: 2–5.

16. Bravo, L. (1998). Polyphenols: chemistry, dietary sources, metabolism, and nutritional significance. *Nutr Rev.* 56: 317–333.

17. Rodríguez, M.L., Estrela, J.M., and Ortega, Á.L. (2013). Natural polyphenols and apop-tosis induction in cancer therapy. *J Carcinogene Mutagene.* S6: 004. doi:10.4172/2157-2518.S6-004.

18. Gutierrez-Merino, C., Lopez-Sanchez, C., Lagoa, R., Samhan-Arias, A.K., and Bueno, C. (2011). Neuroprotective actions of flavonoids. *Curr Med Chem* 18: 1195–1212.

19. Agouni, A., Lagrue-LakHal, A.H., Mostefai, H.A., Tesse, A., and Mulder, P. (2009). Red wine polyphenols prevent metabolic and cardiovascular alterations associated with obesity in Zucker fatty rats (Fa/Fa). *PLoS ONE.* 4: e5557.

20. Burke, A.C., Sutherland, B.G., Telford, D.E., *et al.* (2018). Intervention with citrus flavonoids reverses obesity, and improves metabolic syndrome and atherosclerosis in obese Ldlr-/- mice. *J Lipid Res.* 59(9): 1714–1728.

21. Chen, D., Sun, J., Dong, W., Shen, Y., and Xu, Z. (2018). Effects of polysaccharides and polyphenolics fractions of Zijuan tea (*Camellia sinensis* var. kitamura) on glucosidase activity and blood glucose level and glucose tolerance of hyperglycaemic mice. *Int J Food Sci Tech.* 53(10): 2335–2341. doi: 10.1111/ijfs.13825.

22. Catana, C.S., Atanasov, A.G., and Berindan-Neagoe, I. (2018). Natural products with anti-aging potential: affected targets and molecular mechanisms. *Biotech Adv.* 36(6): 1649–1656. doi: 10.1016/j.biotechadv.2018.03.012

23. Urquiaga, I., and Leighton, F. (2000). Plant polyphenol antioxidants and oxidative stress. *Biol Res.* 33(2), 55–64.

24. Manach, C., Scalbert, A., Morand, C., Rémésy, C., and Jiménez, L. (2004). Polyphenols: food sources and bioavailability. *Am J Clin Nutr.* 79: 727–747.

25. Fulda, S., and Debatin, K.M. (2004). Sensitization for tumor necrosis factor-related apoptosis-inducing ligand-induced apoptosis by the chemopreventive agent resveratrol. *Cancer Res.* 64: 337–346.

26. Huminiecki, L., and Horbanczuk, J. (2018). The functional genomic studies of resveratrol in respect to its anti-cancer effects. *Biotech Adv.* 36(6): Special Issue S1, 1699–1708. Published: Nov 1, 2018

27. Brusselmans, K., De Schrijver, E., Heyns, W., Verhoeven, G., and Swinnen, J.V. (2003). Epigallocatechin-3-gallate is a potent natural inhibitor of fatty acid synthase in intact cells and selectively induces apoptosis in prostate cancer cells. *Int J Cancer.* 106: 856–862.

28. Benitez, D.A., Pozo-Guisado, E., Alvarez-Barrientos, A., Fernandez-Salguero, P.M., and Castellón, E.A. (2007). Mechanisms involved in resveratrol-induced apoptosis and cell cycle arrest in prostate cancer-derived cell lines. *J Androl.* 28: 282–293.

29. Gu, J.J., Qiao, K.S., Sun, P., Chen, P., and Li, Q. (2018). Study of EGCG induced apoptosis in lung cancer cells by inhibiting P13K/Akt signaling pathway. *Eur Rev Med Pharmacol Sci.* 22(14): 4557–4563.

30. Shankar, S., Ganapathy, S., Chen, Q., and Srivastava, R.K. (2008). Curcumin sensitizes TRAIL-resistant xenografts: molecular mechanisms of apoptosis, metastasis and angiogenesis. *Mol Cancer.* 29: 7–16. doi: 10.1186/1476-4598-7-16

31. Chakraborty, A., Gupta, N., Ghosh, K., and Roy, P. (2010). In vitro evaluation of the cytotoxic anti-proliferative and anti-oxidant properties of pterostilbene isolated from Pterocarpus marsupium. *Toxicol In Vitro.* 24: 1215–1228.

32. Lu, G., Xiao, H., You, H., Lin, Y., and Jin, H. (2008). Synergistic inhibition of lung tumorigenesis by a combination of green tea polyphenols and atorvastatin. *Clin Cancer Res.* 14: 4981–4988.

33. Saha, A., Kuzuhara, T., Echigo, N., Suganuma, M., and Fujiki, H. (2010). New role of (-)-epicatechin in enhancing the induction of growth inhibition and apoptosis in human lung cancer cells by curcumin. *Cancer Prev Res (Phila).* 3: 953–962.

34. Khan, N., Adhami, V.M., and Mukhtar, H. (2010). Apoptosis by dietary agents for prevention and treatment of prostate cancer. *Endocr Relat Cancer.* 17: R39–52.

35. Jang, M., Cai, L., Udeani, G.O., *et al.* (1997). Cancer chemopreventive activity of resveratrol, a natural product derived from grapes. *Science.* 275, 218–220. doi: 10.1126/science.275.5297.218.

36. Mena, S., Rodríguez, M.L., Ponsoda, X., Estrela, J.M., Jäättela, M., and Ortega, A.L. (2012). Pterostilbene-induced tumor cytotoxicity: a lysosomal membrane

permeabilization-dependent mechanism. *PLoS ONE.* 7: e44524. doi: 10.1371/journal.pone.0044524.

37. Gokbulut, A.A., Apohan, E., and Baran, Y. (2013). Resveratrol and quercetin-induced apoptosis of human 232B4 chronic lymphocytic leukemia cells by activation of caspase-3 and cell cycle arrest. *Hematology.* 18: 144–150.

38. Frazzi, R., and Tigano, M. (2014).The multiple mechanisms of cell death triggered by resveratrol in lymphoma and leukemia. *Int J Mol Sci.* 15(3): 4977–4993. doi: 10.3390/ijms15034977.

39. Shankar, S., Chen, Q., Siddiqui, I., Sarva, K., and Srivastava, R.K. (2007). Sensitization of TRAIL-resistant LNCaP cells by resveratrol (3, 4′, 5 tri-hydroxystilbene): molecular mechanisms and therapeutic potential. *J Mol Signal.* 2: 7–15.

40. Ivanov, G.S., Ivanova, T., Kurash, J., *et al.* (2007). Methylation-acetylation interplay activates p53 in response to DNA damage. *Mol Cell Biol.* 19: 6756–6769. doi: 10.1128/MCB.00460-07.

41. Lavin, M.F., and Gueven, N. (2006). The complexity of p53 stabilization and activation. *Cell Death Differ.* 13: 941–950.

42. Kapoor, M., Hamm, R., Yan, W., Taya, Y., and Lozano, G. (2000). Cooperative phosphorylation at multiple sites is required to activate p53 in response to UV radiation. *Oncogene.* 19: 358–364.

43. Kai, L., Samuel, S.K., and Levenson, A.S. (2010). Resveratrol enhances p53 acetylation and apoptosis in prostate cancer by inhibiting MTA1/NuRD complex. *Int J Cancer.* 126: 1538–1548.

44. Singh, N., Zaidi, D., Shyam, H., Sharma, R., and Balapure, A.K. (2012). Polyphenols sensitization potentiates susceptibility of MCF-7 and MDA MB-231 cells to centchroman. *PLoS ONE.* 7(6): e37736. doi: 10.1371/journal.pone.0037736.

45. Benitez, D.A., Hermoso, M.A., Pozo-Guisado, E., Fernández-Salguero, P.M., and Castellón, E.A. (2009). Regulation of cell survival by resveratrol involves inhibition of NF kappa B-regulated gene expression in prostate cancer cells. *Prostate.* 69: 1045–1054.

46. Sun, C., Hu, Y., Liu, X., Wu, T., and Wang, Y. (2006). Resveratrol downregulates the constitutional activation of nuclear factor-kappa B in multiple myeloma cells, leading to suppression of proliferation and invasion, arrest of cell cycle, and induction of apoptosis. *Cancer Genet Cytogenet.* 165: 9–19.

47. Gupta, S.C., Patchva, S., Koh, W., and Aggarwal, B.B. (2012). Discovery of curcumin, a component of golden spice, and its miraculous biological activities. *Clin Exp Pharmacol Physiol.* 39: 283–299.

48. Shankar, S., Ganapathy, S., Chen, Q., and Srivastava, R.K. (2008). Curcumin sensitizes TRAIL-resistant xenografts: molecular mechanisms of apoptosis, metastasis and angiogenesis. *Mol Cancer.* 7: 16–23.

49. Adhami, V.M., Siddiqui, I.A., Sarfaraz, S., *et al.* (2009). Effective prostate cancer chemopreventive intervention with green tea polyphenols in the TRAMP model depends on the stage of the disease. *Clin Cancer Res.* 15(6): 1947–1953. doi: 10.1158/1078-0432.CCR-08-2332.

50. Wu, B., Yao, H., Wang, S., and Xu, R. (2013). DAPK1 modulates a curcumin-induced G2/M arrest and apoptosis by regulating STAT3, NF-κB, and caspase-3 activation. *Biochem Biophys Res Commun.* 434: 75–80.

51. McCormack, D., and McFadden, D. (2012). Pterostilbene and cancer: current review. *J Surg Res.* 173, e53–61.
52. Chakraborty, A., Gupta, N., Ghosh, K., and Roy, P. (2010). In vitro evaluation of the cytotoxic, anti-proliferative and anti-oxidant properties of pterostilbene isolated from *Pterocarpus marsupium. Toxicol In Vitro.* 24: 1215–1228.
53. Chen, R.J., Ho, C.T., and Wang, Y.J. (2010). Pterostilbene induces autophagy and apoptosis in sensitive and chemoresistant human bladder cancer cells. *Mol Nutr Food Res.* 54: 1819–1832.
54. Gutierrez, E.M., Seebacher, N.A., Arzuman, L., *et al.* (2016). Lysosomal membrane stability plays a major role in the cytotoxic activity of the anti-proliferative agent, di-2-pyridylketone 4,4-dimethyl-3-thiosemicarbazone (Dp44mT). *Biochim Biophys Acta.* 1863(7 Pt A): 1665–1681. doi: 10.1016/j.bbamcr.2016.04.017.
55. daCosta, D.C.F., Casanova, F.A., Quarti, J., *et al.* (2012). Transient transfection of a wild-type p53 gene triggers resveratrol-induced apoptosis in cancer cells. *PLoS ONE.* 7(11): e48746. doi: 10.1371/journal.pone.0048746.
56. Mannal, P.W., Alosi, J.A., Schneider, J.G., McDonald, D.E., and McFadden, D.W. (2010). Pterostilbene inhibits pancreatic cancer in vitro. *J Gastrointest Surg.* 14: 873–879.
57. Wu, B., Kulkarni, K., Basu, S., Zhang, S., and Hu, M. (2011). First-pass metabolism via UDP-glucuronosyltransferase: a barrier to oral bioavailability of phenolics. *J Pharm Sci.* 100: 3655–3681.
58. Agarwal, A., Kasinathan, A., Ganesan, R., *et al.* (2018). Curcumin induces apoptosis and cell cycle arrest via the activation of reactive oxygen species-independent mitochondrial apoptotic pathway in Smad4 and p53 mutated colon adenocarcinoma HT29 cells. *Nutrition Res.* 51: 67–81. doi: 10.1016/j.nutres.2017.12.011.
59. Lai, H., Wang, Y., Duan, F., *et al.* (2018). Krukovine suppresses KRAS-mutated lung cancer cell growth and proliferation by inhibiting the RAF-ERK pathway and inactivating AKT pathway. *Front Pharmacol.* 9: 958. Published: Aug 22, 2018.
60. Yasuda, H., Sng, N. J., Yeo, W. L., Figueiredo-Pontes, L. L., Kobayashi, S., and Costa, D. (2012). Sensitivity of EGFR exon 20 insertion mutations to EGFR inhibitors is determined by their location within the tyrosine kinase domain of EGFR. *Cancer Res.* 72: 23. doi: 10.1158/1538-7445.AM20 12-23.
61. Heavey, S., O'Byrne, K. J., and Gately, K. (2014). Strategies for co-targeting the PI3K/AKT/mTOR pathway in NSCLC. *Cancer Treat Rev.* 40: 445–456. doi: 10.1016/j.ctrv.2013.08.006.
62. De Grève, J., Teugels, E., Geers, C., Decoster, L., Galdermans, D., and De Mey, J. (2012). Clinical activity of afatinib (BIBW 2992) in patients with lung adenocarcinoma with mutations in the kinase domain of HER2/neu. *Lung Cancer* 76: 123–127. doi: 10.1016/j.lungcan.2012.01.008.
63. Mazières, J., Peters, S., Lepage, B., *et al.* (2012). Lung cancer that harbors an HER2 mutation: epidemiologic characteristics and therapeutic perspectives. *J Clin Oncol.* 31: 1997–2003. doi: 10.1200/JCO.2012.45.6095.
64. Dholwani, K.K., Saluja, A.K., Gupta, A.R., and Shah, D.R.(2008). A review on plant-derived natural products and their analogs with anti-tumor activity. *Indian J Pharmacol.* 40: 49–58.

65. Mostafa, N.M., Ashour, M.L., Eldahshan, O.A., and Singab, A.N.B. (2016). Cytotoxic activity and molecular docking of a novel Bifla-vonoid isolated from *Jacaranda acutifolia* (Bignoniaceae). *Nat Prod Res*. 30: 2093–2100.

66. Al-Sayed, E., Eldahshan, O.A., Bahgat, D.M., and Singab, A.N.B. (2016). Cytotoxic oleanane-type saponins from the leaves of *Albizia anthelmintica* B RONGN. *Chem Biodivers*. 13: 1666–1673

67. Shehzad, A., Lee, J., and Lee, Y.S. (2013). Curcumin in various cancers. *Biofactors*. 39(1): 56–68.

68. Darvesh, A.S., Aggarwal, B.B., and Bishayee, A. (2012). Curcumin and liver cancer: a review. *Curr Pharmaceut Biotechnol*. 13(1): 218–228.

69. Chen, J., Shi, D.Y., Liu, S.L., and Zhong, L. (2012). Tanshinone IIA induces growth inhibition and apoptosis in gastric cancer in vitro and in vivo. *Oncol Reports*. 27(2): 523–528.

70. Ali, R., Mirza, Z., Ashraf, G.M., *et al.* (2012). New anticancer agents: recent developments in tumor therapy. *Anticancer Res*. 32(7): 2999–3005.

71. Chung, J.H., Han, J.H., Hwang, E.J., *et al.* (2003). Dual mechanisms of green tea extract (EGCG)-induced cell survival in human epidermal keratinocytes. *FASEB J*. 17(13): 1913–1915.

72. Mujtaba, T., and Dou, Q.P. (2012). Black tea polyphenols inhibit tumor proteasome activity. *In Vivo*. 26(2): 197–202.

73. Kinjo, J., Morito, K., Tsuchihashi, R., Hirose, T., Aomori, T., and Okawa, M. (2004). Examination for estrogenic activities of soyasaponin I and related compounds. *Nat Med*. 58: 193–197.

74. Ueda, S., Nakamura, H., Masutani, H., *et al.* (2002). Baicalin induces apoptosis via mitochondrial pathway as prooxidant. *Mol Immunol*. 38: 781–791.

75. Abdel-Salam, I., Ashmawy, A.M., Hilal, A., Eldahshan, O.A., and Ashour, M. (2018). Chemical composition of aqueous ethanol extract of luffa cylindrica leaves and its effect on representation of caspase-8, caspase-3, and the proliferation marker Ki67 in intrinsic molecular subtypes of breast cancer in vitro. *Chem Biodivers*. 15(8): 1–13. Article Number: e1800045. doi: 10.1002/cbdv.201800045.

76. Ma, H., Zhou, J., Guo, H., *et al.* (2018). A strategy for the metabolomics-based screening of active constituents and quality consistency control for natural medicinal substance toad venom. *Anal Chim Acta*. 1031: 108–118. doi: 10.1016/j.aca.2018.05.054.

# PHARMACEUTICAL DEVELOPMENT OF POTENTIAL CANCER DRUGS

Medicinal plants have historically shown their value in folk medicine or as a source of new drug and nowadays still represent an important pool for drug development. Traditional Chinese medicine (TCM) has historically been used for thousands of years in China and become alternative medicine in other parts of the world in recent decades. TCM has become a rich source of novel molecules with therapeutic potential. Nowadays, it represents an excellent complementary medicine for treatment of diseases including cancer. Phytochemicals from TCM become an important pool for development of drugs and medical supplements. In the 1990s, pharmaceutical industry focused on libraries of synthetic compounds as a source of drug development. Although established drugs demonstrate pharmacological effects, some of the drugs induce drug toxicity upon regular use in humans. The use of drugs for treatment of cancer may cause serious side effects including neurotoxicity, cardiovascular toxicity, and liver toxicity. However, the combination of phytochemicals with established drugs shows beneficial effects on cancer patients. The adjuvant therapy with cancer drugs has been an increasing trend in cancer therapy. Treatment of diseases with new drugs, which are derived from active phytochemicals, has raised renewed scientific interest in drug discovery from natural sources and herbal medicine.

A recent study has outlined the impact of historical development of drugs and recent developments of plant-derived natural product in drug discovery.[1] The study clearly showed the significant impact of medicinal plants and TCM in drug discovery. Drugs are developed for new treatment strategy for cancer patients.

## Current status of TCM in western medicine

The previous knowledge on the application of medicinal plants in the Western world is mainly based on the Greek and Roman culture.[1] Of particular importance were the compendia written by the Greek physician Dioscorides (first century AD), and by the Romans Pliny the Elder (first century AD) and Galen (second century AD).[2] Medicinal herbs from Chinese and Indian were also recorded.[3] Whereas TCM has historically been used for thousands of years in China and has become increasingly popular in cancer therapy. TCM can be used as adjuvant therapy and adjuvant care. It can be given in addition to the primary cancer therapy with the following health benefits:

(1)  To reduce side effects of drugs
(2)  To enhance efficacy of drugs
(3)  To alleviate pain and sufferings

## Adjuvant cancer therapy

TCM is commonly given as adjuvant treatment after systemic therapy, which includes surgery, for example, breast cancer, chemotherapy, immunotherapy, endocrine therapy, or also known as hormone therapy. Oncologists use statistical methods to assess the cancer risk of disease relapse before deciding on the specific adjuvant therapy. However, detail of statistical analysis of large clinical data on adjuvant treatment with TCM is lacking. Therefore, the statistical evidence to assess the benefits of adjuvant treatment with TCM needs to be established before administration of adjuvant treatment with systemic therapy. The ultimate aim of adjuvant treatment with TCM is to improve cancer-specific complications and overall survival rate. Because the adjuvant treatment is essentially for a risk reduction, it is believed that a proportion of patients who receive adjuvant therapy has already been treated by their primary conventional drug therapy.

Adjuvant systemic therapy and radiotherapy are often given following surgery for common types of cancer, including colon cancer, lung cancer, breast cancer, prostate cancer, and some gynecological cancers. Not all forms of cancer may benefit from adjuvant therapy, however. It is known that certain forms of renal cell carcinoma and brain cancer can benefit from adjuvant therapy with TCM, which can boost the effects of the primary treatments.

## Combination of TCM in complex treatment regimens

The side effects of complex treatment regimens used in conventional cancer therapy have prompted the application of adjuvant therapy with TCM or the phytochemicals in order to ameliorate the undesirable side effects.

The major strength of phytochemical-based drug discovery is the advanced methodology for characterization of various classes of plant-derived phytochemical compounds. However, associated challenges are to determine the mechanism of actions and the respective molecular targets of the potential drug candidate. It would indeed take a long time to establish the statistical evidence of the pharmacological effects of novel phytochemicals before pre-clinical trials of these phytochemical compounds can be performed. Importantly, the transition of a phytochemical compound from a screening test program through a "drug lead" to a "marketed drug" is associated with increasingly challenging demands for both quality and quantity control of the desired compound, which cannot be achieved by extraction of the respective plant sources. In this regard, the existing alternative approach including synthetic preparation of analogues and continuous research into identification of active phytochemicals for drug discovery are warranted.

## Use of ethnopharmacological information in drug discovery

TCM and other medicinal plants have historically been a rich source for drug discovery and still represent an important pool for novel pharmacological agents today. It was reported that renewed scientific interest in herbs-derived phytochemical compounds and natural products-based drug discovery was evident from the analysis of PubMed publication trends.[1] Plants are producing a variety of chemically active secondary metabolites with diverse chemical functionalities. They are the molecular targets to be modified for optimizing biological functions; thus, phytochemicals with multi-arrays of pharmacological activities can be produced; yet they are still far from being exhaustively investigated. Resulting from the fruitful research in natural product-based drug discovery, highly integral approaches with computer-aided algorithms for the identification and characterization of phytochemicals are being developed. One major asset of herbs-based drug discovery is the existence of ethnopharmacological information that provides drug leads for active phytochemicals with therapeutic potential in humans. In order to garner the potential of various phytochemicals, a big data analysis allows more effective drug discovery. The adoption of ethnopharmacological information, phytochemistry, and testing strategies including *in vivo* metabolism and efficacy studies of phytochemicals is necessary. Total chemical synthesis is an effective resupply strategy when needed. Small size potent phytochemicals or natural product derivatives with simple stereo structures are favorable and can be made in a large scale. For complex structures, however, total synthesis remains a challenge and unfavorable in most cases. Although biotechnological production of phytochemicals cannot be applied for industry-scale production at present, it bears potential that can be performed in the future align with the advance knowledge of herbal medicine and their biosynthetic pathways. In addition, the development of genetic engineering strategies in plant metabolism would provide alternate approach to production of desired phytochemicals.

## Interdisciplinary approach to drug discovery

While phytochemicals-based drug discovery and development represent a renewed interest in research of TCM and other medicinal plants, the complexity of research work in TCM demands an integrated interdisciplinary approach to characterize individual phytochemicals. With progress of technologic advances in finger printing of herbal medicine, active phytochemicals can be more readily identified in various classes of medicinal plants. The voluminous literature in herbal medicine suggests that phytochemical compounds remain the most important sources of new drugs. The research trends in drug development clearly reflect the significance of work in phytochemical compounds. The biopharmaceutical industry can boost the economy across China and around the world, which are benefiting from the latest treatments and cures. It is also a highly valuable industry in terms of its economic contributions and impacts. The evolving field of pharmacogenomics (PG), using genomic markers to predict drug response, may impact drug development times, costs, and the future returns.[4] It is known that a major promise of PG is information that can transform health care and risk through earlier diagnosis and implementation of more effective preventive measures and treatment of diseases. More importantly, technologic advances of drug development, which is essentially based on chemistry of phytochemical compounds and their pharmacological activity, can help reduce drug side effects. While there still remains an uncertainty around how PG will help the pharmaceutical industry, there are advantages of PG in drug development. With an established PG program, the expected drug development costs and clinical trials can be significantly reduced. It would improve the cost-effective production of new drugs. The advances of PG would definitely help patients with various diseases and drug resistance in cancer therapy.

A good example of drug development using metabolomics can be demonstrated with natural polyphenols that show multi-arrays of biologic and pharmacologic activities; yet their bioavailability and effectiveness in *in vivo* study seriously limits their development as therapeutics.[4] A combination of metabolomics-based screening and quality consistency control (MSQCC) of active natural polyphenols and their synthetic analogues was shown to provide a practical approach to this long-standing problem.[4] A recent study showed that the screening method offered the co-correlation study of metabolomic and biological profiles of 180 fractions prepared from natural heterogeneous biologic samples as a way to identify a series of bufadinolides as quality control markers for inhibitors of cancer cell.[5] The methodology provides a strategy for a large-scale screening test and application of the control markers in assessment test. The application of metabolomics to *in vivo* study provides information on the metabolic fate of phytochemicals and the half-time of the phytochemicals and their metabolites in the body.

Natural product-based drug discovery has made significant contribution to cancer chemotherapy. It remains an integral part of molecular diversity for anticancer drug discovery. The molecular diversity of phytochemical compounds allows interactions of different molecular targets and to establish palliative strategy for various diseases including cancer. More often than not, active phytochemical compounds may serve as leads for drug development.[6] The transformation of natural leads into anticancer drugs should address the following issues:

(1) Drug efficacy
(2) Optimization of absorption, distribution, metabolism, and excretion (ADME) profiles
(3) Improvement of bioavailability of the natural leads

Optimization strategies for effective drug development involve study of structure–activity relationship of drug candidates. With the advent of computer-aided drug design and big data analysis, novel drug can be readily developed.

In recent years, many excellent review articles have highlighted the contributions of natural products to drug discovery.[7-9] Other reports emphasized the influence of phytochemicals on the discovery of new chemical entities and active functionalities that are involved in the respective biologic activities including signaling processes related to cancer growth and metastasis.[10-13] Although TCM remains an indispensable source of molecular and mechanistic diversity for anticancer drug discovery, the number of anticancer phytochemicals that can be transformed to clinical drugs remains low. However, active phytochemicals provide insight into drug development rather than as effective anticancer drugs by themselves.

## Economic impact of natural products and phytochemicals

It was reported that during the time period from 1981 to 2010, when all the approved small size drugs categorized as either a new **drug product** or as a new **drug substance** are considered, only 36% of them are synthetic molecules.[13] The rest of pharmaceutical products was originated from natural products. The study showed natural products played an important role in the drug discovery. They are more important for lead identification and drug discovery in cancer therapy.[14,15] The percentage of natural product-based molecules in anticancer drugs is significantly higher than in average drugs with 79.8% for anticancer drugs approved in 1981–2010 and 74.9% for all the anticancer drugs approved worldwide.[13] The significant impact of natural products in cancer drug discovery was reported before[16-20] and in the recent years.[1,21,22] Phytochemicals-based drug discovery bears substantial impact on health and economy across countries all over the world.

# Breakthroughs in immunotherapy

The Nobel Prize in Physiology or Medicine 2018 was awarded jointly to James P. Allison and Tasuku Honjo for their discovery of cancer therapy by inhibition of negative immune regulation and modulation of CTLA-4 and PD-1 activity resulting in activation of T cells to fight against cancer. The immune response can be modulated by drugs and natural products. The two scientists were honored for their pioneering work in immunotherapy, which harnesses the body's immune system to attack cancer.

Their work has "revolutionized cancer treatment" and is "a landmark in our fight against cancer," the Nobel Assembly said.

The way we treat cancer is about to change forever. This revolution was sparked not by the invention of a new drug but by the evolution of an entirely new way of thinking about modulation of immune response and cancer therapy. Going forward, doctors will not only use pharmaceuticals to attack tumors. Rather, the oncologist will treat the patient's immune system with a drug or specific natural products for managing cancer.

It's a peek into the potential of herbal medicine and other natural products and thoughts of combination of drugs and herbal medicine in immunotherapy for various diseases. The discovery in herbal medicine for cancer therapy would show readers the many decades of devotion and passion it takes to imagine a better world and then to make it happen. If this book motivates more talented and visionary investigators to devote more efforts in research in herbal medicine for immunotherapy, it would be a wonderful success.

# References

1. Atanasov, A.G., Waltenberger, B., Pferschy-Wenzig, E.M., *et al.* (2015). Discovery and resupply of pharmacologically active plant-derived natural products: a review. *Biotechnol. Adv.* 33(8): 1582–1614. doi: 10.1016/j.biotechadv.2015.08.001.
2. Sneader, W. (2005). *Drug Discovery: a History*. New Jersey, US, Wiley.
3. Cragg, G.M., and Newman, D.J. (2013). Natural products: a continuing source of novel drug leads. *Biochim. Biophys. Acta.* 1830: 3670–3695.

4. Simonds, N.I., Khoury, M.J., Schully, S.D., *et al.* (2013).Comparative effectiveness research in cancer Genomics and precision medicine: current landscape and future prospects. *J Nat Can Institute.* 105(13): 929–936. doi: 10.1093/jnci/djt108.

5. Ma, H., Zhou, J., Guo, H., *et al.* (2018). A strategy for the metabolomics-based screening of active constituents and quality consistency control for natural medicinal substance toad venom. *Anal Chim Acta.* 1031: 108–118. Published: November 15, 2018.

6. Xiao, Z., Morris-Natschke, S.L., and Lee, K.H. (2016). Strategies for the optimization of natural leads to anticancer drugs or drug candidates. *Med Res Rev.* 36(1): 32–91. doi: 10.1002/med.21377.

7. Kinghorn, A.D., Pan, L., Fletcher, J.N., and Chai, H. (2011).The relevance of higher plants in lead compound discovery programs. *J Nat Prod.* 74: 1539–1555.

8. Mishra, B.B., and Tiwari, V.K. (2011). Natural products: an evolving role in future drug discovery. *Eur J Med Chem.* 46: 4769–4807.

9. Cragg, G.M., and Newman, D.J. (2013). Natural products: a continuing source of novel drug leads. *Biochim Biophys Acta.* 1830: 3670–3695.

10. Cragg, G.M., Newman, D.J., and Snader, K.M. (1997). Natural products in drug discovery and development. *J Nat Prod.* 60: 52–60.

11. Newman, D.J., Cragg, G.M., and Snader, K.M. (2003). Natural products as sources of new drugs over the period 1981–2002. *J Nat Prod.* 66: 1022–1037.

12. Newman, D.J., and Cragg, G.M. (2007). Natural products as sources of new drugs over the last 25 years. *J Nat Prod.* 70: 461–477.

13. Newman, D.J., and Cragg, G.M. (2012). Natural products as sources of new drugs over the 30 years from 1981 to 2010. *J Nat Prod.* 75: 311–335.

14. Butler, M.S. (2008). Natural products to drugs: natural product-derived compounds in clinical trials. *Nat Prod Rep.* 25: 475–516.

15. Shu, Y.Z. (1998). Recent natural products based drug development: a pharmaceutical industry perspective. *J Nat Prod.* 61: 1053–1071.

16. Das, B., and Satyalakshmi, G. (2012). Natural products based anticancer agents. *Mini-Rev Org Chem.* 9: 169–177.

17. Gordaliza, M. (2007). Natural products as leads to anticancer drugs. *Clin Transl Oncol.* 9: 767–776.

18. Cragg, G.M., Grothaus, P.G., and Newman, D.J. (2009). Impact of natural products on developing new anticancer agents. *Chem Rev.* 109: 3012–3043.

19. Salvador, J.A.R., Carvalho, J.F.S., Neves, M.A.C., *et al.* (2013). Anticancer steroids: linking natural and semi-synthetic compounds. *Nat Prod Rep.* 30: 324–374.

20. Cragg, G.M., Kingston, D.G.I., and Newman, D.J. eds. (2011). *Anticancer Agents from Natural Products.* 2. London, CRC Press, Taylor & Francis Group.

21. Zhang, B., Peng, Y., Zhang, Z., *et al.* (2010). GAP production of TCM herbs in China. *Planta Med.* 76(17): 1948–55. doi: 10.1055/s-0030-1250527.

22. Chen, X., Pei, L., and Lu, J. (2013). Filling the gap between traditional Chinese medicine and modern medicine, are we heading to the right direction? *Complement Ther Med.* 21(3): 272–275. doi: 10.1016/j.ctim.2013.01.001.

(chemical structures of phytochemical compounds. The reactive moiety/ atom are highlighted in color.)

# Chapter 2

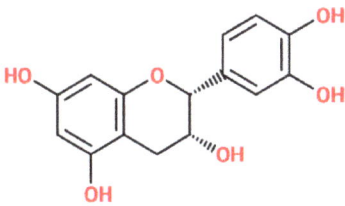

(-)-epicatechin

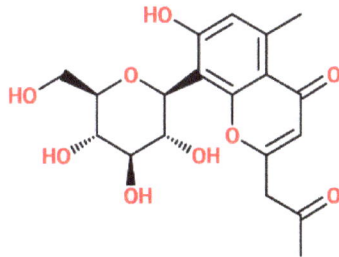

aloesin

**Anacardic acid**

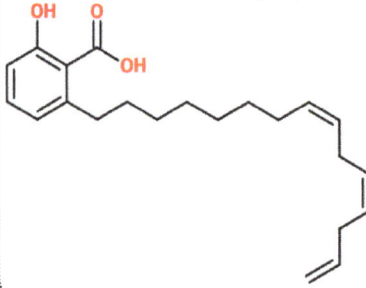

**argentilactone**

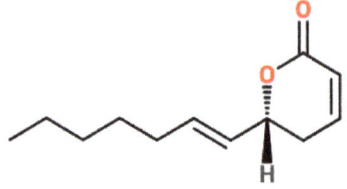

**Caffeic acid**

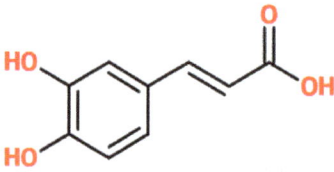

**Diosgenin**

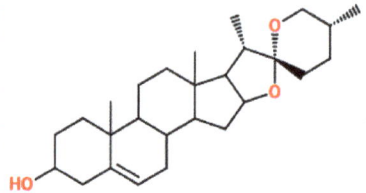

**Eugenol**

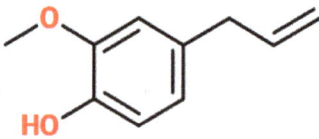

**Ferulic acid**

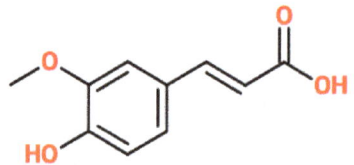

## gallic acid

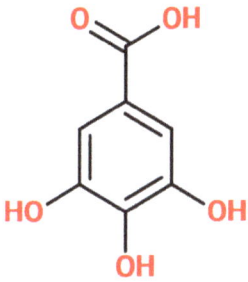

## Genistein

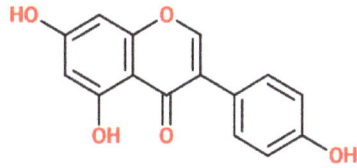

## Glucobrassicin

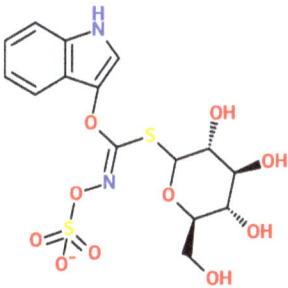

## Glycyrrhetinic acid

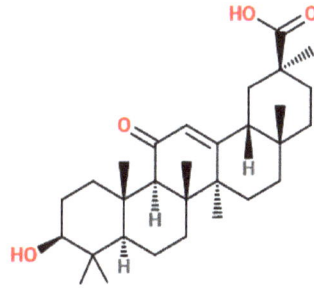

## Harmine

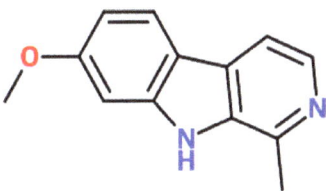

## isotetradrine

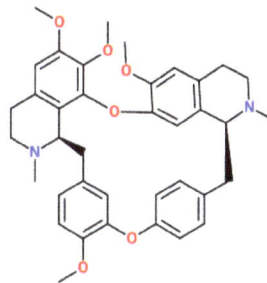

## Luteolin

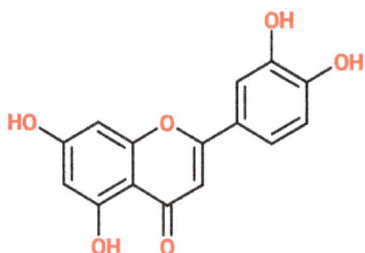

## Nobiletin

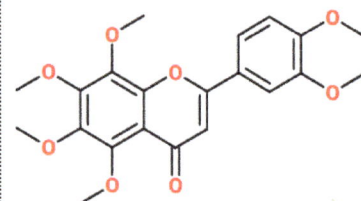

## Paeonol

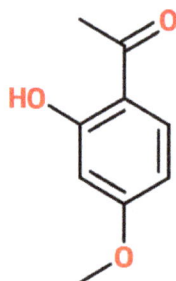

## Phelligridins D

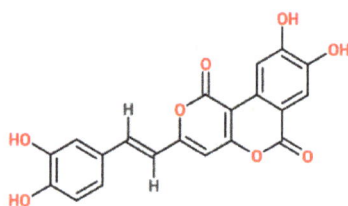

## Pomiferin

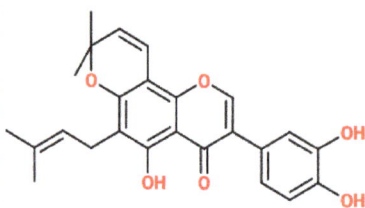

## Pomolic acid

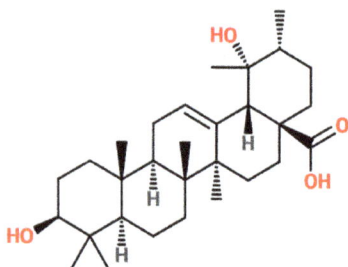

## Rooperol

## rosmarinic acid

## scopoletin

## sulphoraphane

## theophylline

## Tocotrienol

## Verbascoside

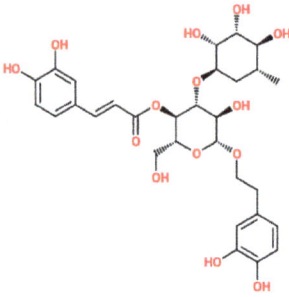

## Wogonin

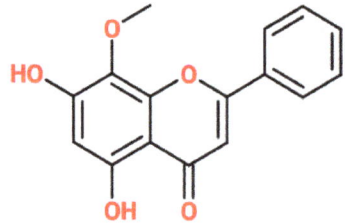

# Chapter 5

## 6-methylsulfinyl hexyl isothiocyanate

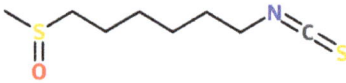

## Ajoene

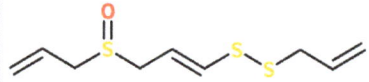

## Allicin

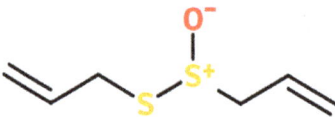

## diallyl sulfide

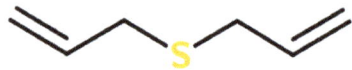

**diallyl trisulfide**

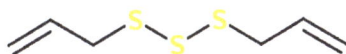

**S-allylmercaptocysteine**

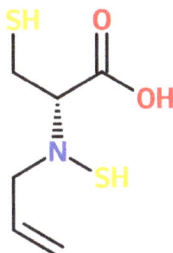

**Sulforaphane**

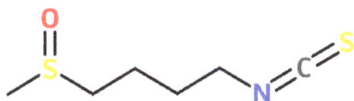

# Chapter 7

**actinodaphnine**

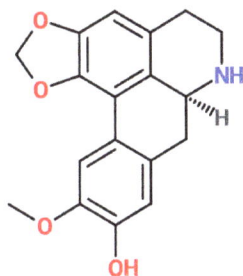

**Apratoxin A**

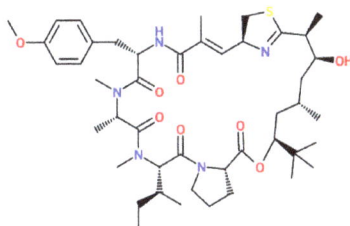

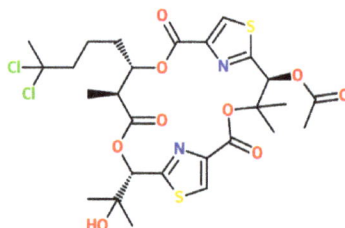

**boldine**

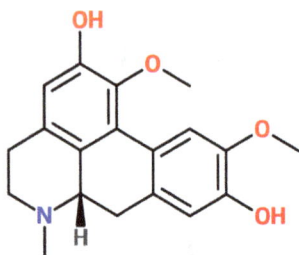

**Camptothecin**

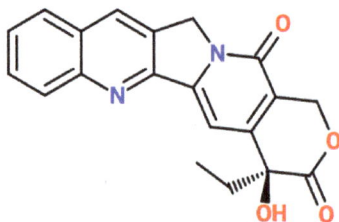

**Dicentrine**

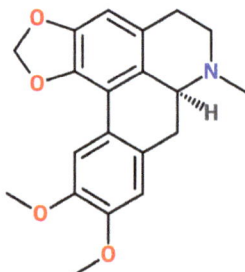

**hectochlorin**

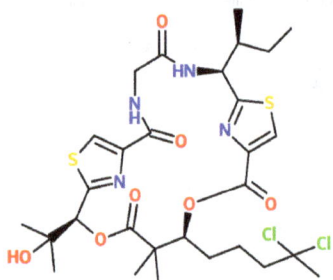

**lyngbyabellin A**

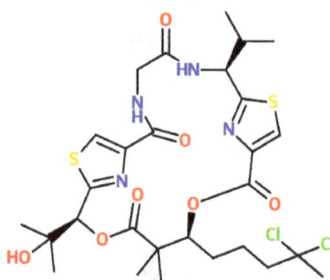

**lyngbyabellin B**

## Piperine

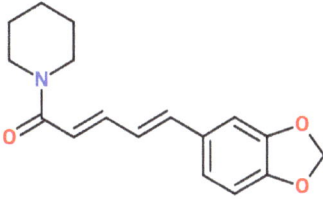

## Piplartine

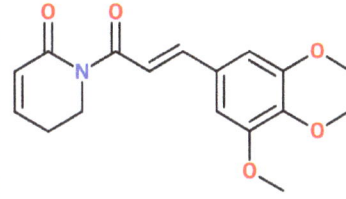

# Chapter 9

## 4,5-dimethylresorcinol

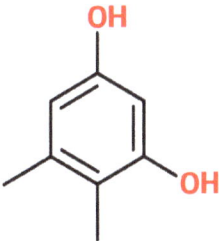

## 4-ethylguaiacol

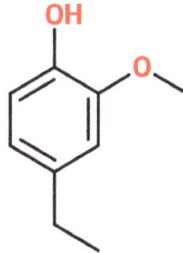

## alliin

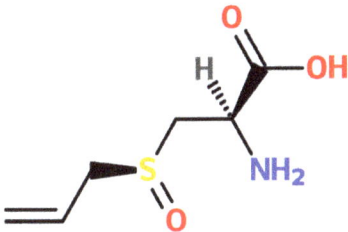

## apigenin 7,4'-dimethyl ether

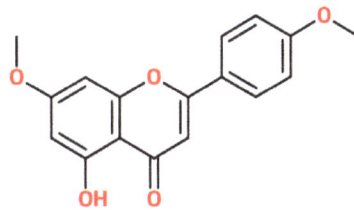

**caffeine**

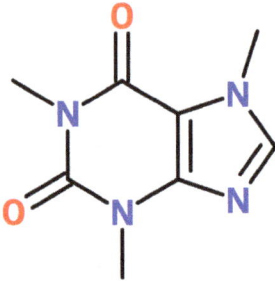

**carvacrol**

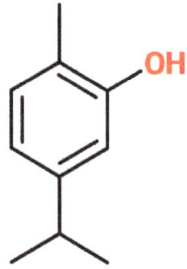

**cathinone**

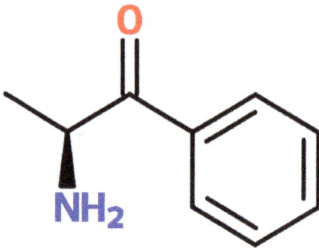

**Coumarin**

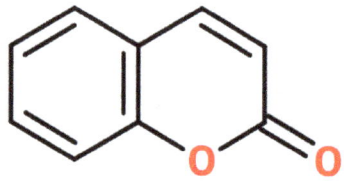

**creosol**

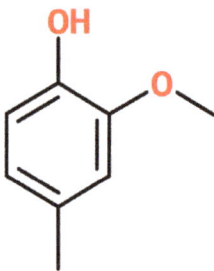

**guaiacol**

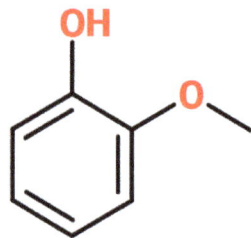

## hyperforin

## hypericin

## kaempferol 7,4'-dimethyl ether

## o-cresol

## p-cresol

## piperine

**quercitrin**

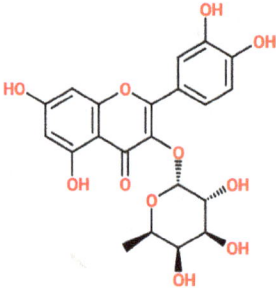

**sakuranetin**

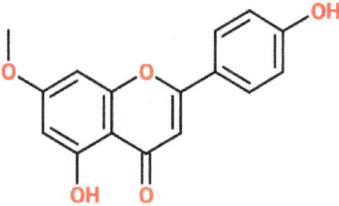

**ternatin**

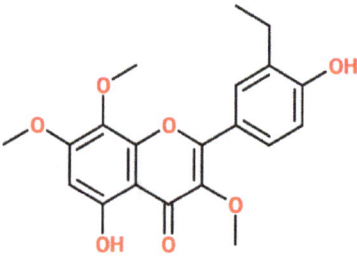

A549 lung cells, 76
KB16 cells, 76
K562 cells, 78
K562/DNR cells, 110
p53, 52
  acetylation, 113
  activation, 43
  mediated expression, 43
  regulates, 52, 55
  tumor suppressor gene, 43
P388 leukemia, 76

## A

ABCB1 transporter, 109–110
abnormal cell growth, 48
*Acacia nilotica*, 91
acerinol, 110
*N*-acetylation, 79
acetyl-coenzyme A, 87
*N*-acetylcysteine (NAC), 19
aconitum alkaloids, 99
*Aconitum carmichaelii*, 99
ACSOs. *See* alk(en)yl cysteine
  sulfoxides
actinodaphnine, 83
  chemical structures, 137

active phytochemicals, 1
  with sulfhydryl (R–SH) group,
    55–57
activity-based fractionation, of TCM
  extracts, 31–32
acupuncture, for cancer treatment,
  11–12
acute kidney injury, 101–102
ADEs. *See* adverse drug events
adjuvant cancer therapy, 124–125
ADM. *See* adriamycin
adriamycin (ADM), 108–109
ADRs. *See* adverse drug reactions
ADT. *See* androgen-deprivation
  therapy
adverse drug events (ADEs), 100
adverse drug reactions (ADRs), 96, 103
  anti-epileptics, 102
  anti-infective agents, 102
  cellular activity, 98–99
  in children, 102
  compressed sensing, 104
  drug toxicity of doxorubicin, 103
  effects of antibiotics and, 99–100
  harmful effects of, 96–97
  incidence rates for, 102

management, 97–98
morbidity and mortality, 100
multiple medications, 97
novel compounds, 103–104
prevalence and characteristics, 98
reduction of, 97
time dependent, 97
aglycone diosgenin, 1, 17
aglycones, 16–17
AIDS, 2
ajoene, 57
chemical structures, 136
AKT inhibitors, 115
Alkaloids, 70, 76
*S*-alkaloids, 79
alk(en)yl cysteine sulfoxides
(ACSOs), 93
allicin, 57
chemical structures, 136
alliin, chemical structures, 139
Allison, James P., 129
*Allium cepa*, 88–89, 93
*Allium* species, flavonoids in, 93
allopathic medicines, 64
*S*-allylmercaptocysteine, 56
chemical structures, 137
aloesin, 26
chemical structures, 131
*Ampelocera edentula*, 18
anacardic acid (6-pentadecylsalicylic
acid), 25
chemical structures, 132
ancient complex therapy theory, 9
ancient herbal formulation, 35
androgen-deprivation therapy (ADT),
97–98
angiogenesis, 34
annona species (Annonaceae), 98
anthocyanidins, 4
anti-angiogenesis, 1
anti-angiogenic herbs, 34
anti-apoptotic signaling events, 54
antiatherogenic herbal compounds, 8

anticancer activities, 76–77
ayurvedic medicinal plant with, 19
of *Glycyrrhiza uralensis* (licorice),
44–46
of plant extracts and fractions, 18–19
anticancer compounds, 81
screening test for, 18
anticancer drugs, 12, 69, 70, 76, 128
natural products as, 115–117
potential, 44
proteinaceous, 43
sources of recombinant, 43–44
anti-cancer herbs, 11
anti-cancer phytochemicals, health
benefits of, 6
antimicrobial activities, 42
anti-obesity drugs, 87
antioxidant, 42
activity, 9
antioxidant response elements
(AREs), 45
antipsychotics, 97
anti-tumor agents drugs, 52
anti-tumorigenic activity of chrysin, 43
anti-tumorigenic effects, 1
apigenin 7,4'-dimethyl ether, chemical
structures, 139
apoptosis, 17, 19, 47
p53 regulates, 52
c-Myc, role of, 54–55
cross-talk among signaling
pathways in, 50
death receptor pathway, 48–49, 50
deregulation of, 48
extrinsic pathway, 48–49
intrinsic pathway of, 49, 52
microRNAs in, 52–53
mitochondrial pathway, 49
modulation of, 51–52
and necrosis, 50
NF-jB in, 52
regulators of, 51
through caspases, regulation of, 54

apoptotic peptidase activating factor-1(Apaf-1), 49, 51
aporphines, 76–77, 79
  cytotoxic actions of, 78–79
aporphines *S*-ovigerine, 76
aporphinoids, 75, 76
  role of, 75–76
apratoxin A, 82
  chemical structures, 137
*Arctotis arctotoides* (L.f.), 42
AREs. *See* antioxidant response
  elements
argentilactone, 22
  chemical structures, 132
*Artemisia annua,* 34
*Ascophyllum nodosum,* 92
aspartate transaminase (AST), 45
aspartic acid proteases, 47
AST. *See* aspartate transaminase
Atg13, 53
ATGs. *See* autophagy-related genes
atherogenesis, 8
atherosclerosis, herbal medicines for
  treatment, 8
ATM-Chk2 pathway, 43
aurilides, 82
autophagy, 49
  cross-talk among signaling
    pathways in, 50
  pathways in cancer, 53
autophagy-related genes (ATGs), 49
avicins, 17
ayurvedic medicinal plant, 19


**B**

baicalin, 34, 116
balanitin-6, 116
balanitin-7, 116
BB. *See* bioavailability barrier
Bcl-2family, 51, 52
*Begonia pearcei,* 18

benzylisoquinoline alkaloids, 77
berberine (BBR), 68
berries, 92
beta-elemene, 110
big data analysis, 69
bioactive alkaloid, 68
bioactive anti-HSV molecules, 3
bioactive compounds, 42, 45
  functional food with, 92
  in seaweed, 92
bioavailability barrier (BB), 99
bioinformatics, 32, 35, 67, 68
biomarkers, 35
biorefineries, 92
biotechnology, 34
bisphosphonate (BP), 101
blood circulation, 11
blueberries, 89–90
*Bocconia integrifolia,* 18
body functions, harmony of, 10
boldine, 83
  chemical structures, 138
BP. *See* bisphosphonate
breast cancer, 53, 100, 117
broccoli, 5
brusatol, 98–99
bufadinolide, 117
bulbocapnine, 79
*S*-bulbocapnine, 79


**C**

caffeic acid, 24
  chemical structures, 132
caffeine, chemical structures, 140
caloric restriction (CR), 111
calorie restriction mimetics
  (CRM), 111
CAM. *See* complementary and
  alternative medicine
*Camellia sinensis,* 34
*Camptotheca acuminata,* 76

camptothecin (CPT), 76, 82
  chemical structures, 138
cancer, 48. *See also* cancer therapy
  ancient herbal formulation, 35
  autophagic pathways in
    Atg13, 53
    PI3KCI-AKT-mTORC1, 53
    ULK1/2, 53
  autophagy and, 49
  biology, 35
  complications, 18
  development of, 11
  diet for, 32
  immune deficiency, 17
  metastasis of, 17
  microRNA–mRNA profiles, 68
  molecular mechanism of, 48–49
  necrosis and, 49–50
  signaling pathways in, 50
  therapy, 18
  treatment, acupuncture for, 11–12
cancer therapy, 30, 107. *See also* cancer
  bisphosphonate use in, 101
  cytotoxic phytochemical
    compounds in, 80–83
  economic impact of, 107
  effects of chloroquine, 101–102
  phytochemicals and phytotherapy
    in, 68–69
  traditional Chinese Medicine
    formulations in, 63
CARD. *See* caspase recruitment
  domain
carvacrol, chemical structures, 140
caspase-9, 51
caspase recruitment domain
  (CARD), 51
caspases, 47, 49
  activator of, 51, 54
*Cassytha filiformis* (Lauraceae), 78
cassythine, 83
cathinone, chemical structures, 140
CDK2. *See* cyclin-dependent kinase-2

cell-based screening method, 43
cell cycle arrest, 17
cell death, 47
  autophagic, 49
  distinctive types of, 48
cellular response, 69
*Ceratonia siliqua*, 91
chemical structures, of phytochemical
  compounds, 131–142
chemical synthesis, 126
chemical technology, 34
chemo-informatics, 32
chemotherapy, 33, 34
  drawback with, 70
  protocols, 69
children, adverse drug reactions in, 102
Chinese herbal medicines, 8, 12, 65
Chinese medical therapies, 67
Chinese medicine (CM), 9–12, 62, 63,
  65–66
  as chronotherapy against cancer, 66
  supportive cancer care, 67
Chinese proprietary medicine, 61
Chinese traditional medicine. *See*
  traditional Chinese medicine
chlorogenic acid, chemical
  properties, 33
chloroquine, 101–102
*Chondrus crispus*, 92
chromosomal translocations, 70
chronic disease, 17
chrysin, anti-tumorigenic activity of, 43
CI. *See* combination index
*Cimicifuga acerina*, 109
cisplatin, 102
*Clostridium difficile*, 97
CM. *See* Chinese medicine
c-Myc
  overexpression of, 55
  proto-oncogene, 54
  role of, 54–55
  target genes of, 54
colonic microflora, 92

combination index (CI), 31
common cancer therapy, 11
complementary and alternative
    medicine (CAM), 64, 65, 67
complex treatment regimens, 125
"compressed sensing" (CS), 104
consciousness, loss of, 96
convulsions, 96
*Corydalis yanhusuo,* 108
S-corydine, 77
costunolide, 19–21
coumarin, chemical structures, 140
CR. *See* caloric restriction
o-cresol, chemical structures, 141
p-cresol, chemical structures, 141
CRISPR/Cas9 platform, 43
CRM. *See* calorie restriction mimetics
cruciferous vegetables, 5–8
*Curcuma aromatica,* 31
*Curcuma longa,* 34, 114
*Curcuma wenyujin,* 110
curcumin, 31–32, 111, 114, 116
cyclin-dependent kinase-2(CDK2), 44
cyclooxygenase, 113
Cyclosporine, 19
cynaropicrin, 19, 21
CYP3A. *See* cytochrome P450 family
    3subfamily A
cysteine, 47
cytochrome *c,* 49, 51
cytochrome P450 family 3subfamily A
    (CYP3A), 45
cytogenetics, 70
cytostatic effects, *saussurea costus,* 20
cytotoxic activities, 76–77
    aporphines, 78–79
    isoquinoline alkaloids, 79
    spirostanol saponin, 80
    *Stephania pierrei,* 79
cytotoxic drugs, side effects, 71–72
cytotoxic phytochemical compounds,
    80–83
cytotoxic plant molecules, 75

**D**

daidzein, 17
danshen. *See Salvia miltiorrhiza*
Danzhi Xiaoyao powder (DXP), 101
DDAs. *See* diester-diterpene alkaloids
DDIs. *See* drug–drug interactions
death effector domain (DED), 50
Death-inducing signaling complex
    (DISC), 48, 50
death receptor (DR) pathway,
    48–50, 54
DED. *See* death effector domain
dehydrocostus lactone (DL), 19, 20
dehydroxyrooperol I, 24
dehydroxyrooperol II, 24
de novo lipogenesis, 87
diabetes mellitus (DM), 88
diallyl sulfide, 56
    chemical structures, 136
diallyl trisulfide, 56
    chemical structures, 137
dicentrine, 79, 83
    chemical structures, 138
S-dicentrine, 78, 79
diester-diterpene alkaloids (DDAs), 99
diet, 5, 32
dietary flavonoids, in healthcare
    products, 88
4,5-dimethylresorcinol, chemical
    structures, 139
dioscin, 1, 17–18, 25
diosgenin, 26
    chemical structures, 132
dipalmitoylphosphatidylcholine/
    dipalmitoylphosphatidylglycerol
    (DPPC/DPPG), 41
DISC. *See* Death-inducing signaling
    complex
DL. *See* dehydrocostus lactone
DM. *See* diabetes mellitus
DMEs. *See* drug-metabolizing
    enzymes

DNA, 72
dose administered, time course, and
    susceptibility (DoTS), 96
DoTS. *See* dose administered, time
    course, and susceptibility
doxorubicin, 103
DPPC/DPPG. *See*
    dipalmitoylphosphatidylcholine/
    dipalmitoylphosphatidylglycerol
drug
    cytotoxicity, 30
    doses, 97
    metabolism of, 96
    product, 128
    resistance, 69, 107–108
    safety in humans, 96
    substance, 128
    toxicity, 69, 97
        of doxorubicin, 103
drug development
    optimization strategies for, 128
    using metabolomics, 127
drug discovery
    ethnopharmacological information
        use in, 125–126
    herbs-based, 126
    interdisciplinary approach to,
        126–128
    natural product-based, 127
    phytochemicals based, 126, 129
drug–drug interactions (DDIs), 98, 102
drug-metabolizing enzymes (DMEs),
    55, 99
    polymorphisms of, 99


**E**

EBM. *See* evidence-based medicine
Ebola diseases, 2
Echinatin, 45
efflux transporters (ETs), 99

EGCG. *See*
    (-)-epigallocatechin-3-gallate
11 cell- and enzyme-based bioassay
    methods, 44
emodin, 33
(-)-epicatechin, 24
    chemical structures, 131
(-)-epigallocatechin-3-gallate (EGCG),
    111, 112, 116
Epstein–Barr virus, 79
ER-positive breast cancer, 101
ethanol extract, *Stephania pierrei*
    (Menispermaceae), 79
ethno-medical knowledge, 18
ethnopharmacological information, in
    drug discovery, 125–126
4-ethylguaiacol, chemical
    structures, 139
eugenol, 24
    chemical structures, 132
eukaryotic cell cycle, 44
evidence-based medicine (EBM),
    62, 66
extrinsic pathway, 48–49


**F**

FADD. *See* Fas-associated death
    domain
Fas-associated death domain (FADD),
    48, 50, 54
ferulic acid, 27
    chemical structures, 132
flavan-3-ols, 4
flavonoids, 3–5, 88
    in *Allium* species, 93
    anti-cancer activities, 5
    common plant, 4
    in healthcare products, 92–93
flavonols, 4
flow cytometry, 31

fluorescence analysis, 31
food supplements, 32
Fourier-transform infrared
    (FTIR), 41
frozen shoulder, 62
Fructus Bruceae, 98
fruit pods, 91
FTIR. *See* Fourier-transform infrared
*Fucus* sp., 92
functional food, with bioactive
    compounds, 92
Fuzi, 99

# G

*Galipea longiflora,* 18
gallic acid, 26
    chemical structures, 133
gambierol, 27
*Ganoderma lingzhi,* 37
*Garcinia cambogia,* 87
*Garcinia gummi-gutta,* 87
*Garcinia mangostana,* 91
garlic, 93
gastric cancer, 20
GBS. *See* glucobrassicin
gene-based drug development, 3
gene editing systems, 43
gene expression profile, 31
gene ontology, 68
generally recognized as safe
    (GRAS), 114
genetic aberrations, 71
genetic engineering, 126
genistein
    chemical structures, 133
    plasma concentration of, 17
*Ginkgo biloba,* 34
ginseng, 12
ginsenosides (dammaranes), 1, 17, 25
glaucine, 108

S-glaucine, 79
glucagon-like peptide-1(GLP-1), 97
glucobrassicin (GBS), 26
    chemical structures, 133
glucose- 6-phosphate
    dehydrogenase, 97
glucosides, 16, 17
glucosinolates, 5
    in cruciferous vegetables, 6
    in human gastrointestinal tract, 5
    hydrolysis products, 6
18β-glycyrrhetinic acid, 45
P-glycoprotein (P-gp), 12, 99, 108, 110
glycyrrhetinic acid, 23
    chemical structures, 133
*Glycyrrhiza uralensis* (licorice), 33,
    44–46
glycyrrhizic acid, 45, 46
goitrin, 6
*Gracilaria* sp., 92
grape polyphenols, 89
GRAS. *See* generally recognized as safe

# H

harmine, 25
    chemical structures, 133
HCA. *See* hydroxycitric acid
HDIs. *See* herb–drug interactions
health benefits, of herbal medicines, 31
healthcare products
    dietary flavonoids in, 88
    flavonoids in, 92–93
    herbal medicine for, 87
    phenolics in, 92–93
    with plant extracts, 90–91
    with sulfur compounds, 88–89
heat shock protein 70(HSP70), 115
hectochlorin, 82
    chemical structures, 138
HeLa. *See* human cervical carcinoma

hemolysis, 97
hepatocellular carcinoma (HCC), 98
hepatoma cell line (HepG2), 110
hepatotoxicity, 86
HepG2. *See* human liver carcinoma
herbaceous infusions, 8
herbal extracts, 32, 33
   chemical components, 80
   quality assurance of, 33
herbal formulations, 34
   in ameliorating drug toxicity, 101
   effects of, 32–33
   traditional, 33
   usage of, 35
herbal medicine-derived compounds, 3
herbal medicines, 1, 2, 30, 32–33, 36,
   42, 129
   advantages, 34
   for atherosclerosis treatment, 8
   for cardiovascular diseases, 8
   Chinese, 8
   clinical evaluation of, 33–36
   co-administration of, 64–65
   evidence-based validation of, 87
   exploitation and use, 6
   in food supplements, 32
   health benefits of, 31
   lucidumol C, 37
   physcion-8-*O*-β-d-monoglucoside,
     37–39
   phytochemicals in, 1
   rich source for drug development,
     30–31
   saponins in, 16
   tamaractam, 36
   traditional Chinese medicine. *See*
     traditional Chinese medicine
   use of, 97
herbal mixtures, 69
herbal plants, 43
herbal products
   consumption of, 86
   development process, 86

herb–drug interactions (HDIs),
   64, 99
herbs, 18, 108
*Hernandia nymphaeifolia*
   (Hernandiaceae), 76
HJD. *See* Huanglian Jiedu Decoction
HL-60 human leukemia cells, 19, 20
Honjo, Tasuku, 129
hormone-sensitive cancers, 6
*Houttuynia cordata* Thunb, 41–42
HSP70. *See* heat shock protein 70
HT-29 colon cells, 76
Huanglian Jiedu Decoction
   (HJD), 67
human cancer cells, 37
human cervical carcinoma (HeLa), 37
human colorectal carcinoma, 37
human intestinal bacteria, myrosinase
   activity of, 5
human liver carcinoma (HepG2), 37
human umbilical vein endothelial cells
   (HUVECs), 21
HUVECs. *See* human umbilical vein
   endothelial cells
hydroperoxidase, 113
hydroxycitric acid (HCA), 87
hyperforin, chemical structures, 141
hypericin, chemical structures, 141
hypothyroidism, 6

**I**

IBS. *See* irritable bowel syndrome
immune deficiency, cancer, 17
immunopharmacology, 75
immunotherapy, 129
individual medicine, 68
indole glucosinolates, 6
infectious diseases, 2
inflammation, 42
interdisciplinary approach, drug
   discovery, 126–128

intrinsic pathway, 49, 52
*in vitro* models, 42
*in vivo* models, 42
irritable bowel syndrome
(IBS), 61
isobologram, 31
*S*-isocorydine, 77
isoflavones, 16
plasma concentration of, 17
isolated compounds, 107
isoquinoline cytotoxicity, 77
isotetradrine, chemical
structures, 133
isotetrandrine, 22
isothiocyanates, 5
iyngbyabellin A, 138
iyngbyabellin B, 138

**J**

*Jacaranda acutifolia,* 116
jaceosidin, 33
JAKs. *See* Janus kinases
Janus kinases (JAKs), 72
Japanese herbal medicine, 62

**K**

kaempferol-apigenin, 116
kaempferol 7,4'-dimethyl ether,
chemical structures, 141
Kampo, 62
KDR/Flk-1, 21
KEGG pathways. *See* Kyoto
Encyclopedia of Genes and
Genomes pathways
KRAS gene, 115
krukovine, 115
Kyoto Encyclopedia of Genes and
Genomes (KEGG) pathways,
67, 68

**L**

*Laminaria* sp., 92
lappadilactone, 20
large molecule drugs, 81
LDL. *See* low-density lipoprotein
LDL-C. *See* LDL cholesterol
LDL cholesterol (LDL-C), 92–93
lean tissue depletion, 103
*Leishmania amazonesis,* 18
let-7family, 52
licorice, 44–46
lignans, 76
*Lindera megaphylla* (Lauraceae), 78
lipid membranes, 41
lipoprotein cholesterol, 89
liraglutide, 98
*Lithospermum officinale,* 86
loss of consciousness, 96
low-density lipoprotein (LDL), 92
lucidumol C, 37
luciferase reporter assay, 45
*Luffa cylindrica,* 117
luminescence, 36
luteolin, 23
chemical structures, 134
lyngbyabellins, 82

**M**

*S*-magnoflorine, 76
*Magnolia officinalis,* 34
magnolol, 33
malignant cells, 112
mall molecule drugs, 81
MAPK. *See* mitogen-activated protein
kinase
MCF7 cells, 43
MDR. *See* multidrug resistance
medicinal herbs, 70
medicinal plants, 9, 75, 123–126
phytochemicals of, 44

melanoma A375, 33
metabolomics-based screening
and quality consistency control
(MSQCC), 117, 127
metabolomics, drug development
using, 127
N-methylation, 79
S-methylcysteine, 88
S-N-methylovigerine, 76
6-methylsulfinyl hexyl
isothiocyanate, 56
chemical structures, 136
microRNAs (miRNAs),
52–53, 68
MiR-34 family, 52
miRNA-21, 52–53
mitochondrial outer membrane
permeability (MOMP), 50, 51
mitochondrial pathway, 49, 51
mitochondrial permeability transition
(MPT), 19
mitogen-activated protein kinase
(MAPK), 72, 110
mitostatic drug paclitaxel (Taxol), 43
mitoxantrone, 108
Molecular Operating Environment
(MOE v2009) software, 44
MOMP. *See* mitochondrial outer
membrane permeability
monoclonal antibodies, 71
*Moringa oleifera*, 91
MPT. *See* mitochondrial permeability
transition
mRNA, 68
MRP. *See* multidrug resistance-
associate protein
MRP1. *See* multidrug resistance-
associate protein 1
MRP2. *See* multidrug resistance-
associated protein 2
MSQCC. *See* metabolomics-based
screening and quality consistency
control

multidrug resistance (MDR), 32,
108–110
multidrug resistance-associated
protein 2(MRP2), 99
multidrug resistance-associate protein
1(MRP1), 108
multidrug resistance-associate protein
(MRP), 108–109
multi-protein complex, 51
muscle loss, 103
mutations, of growth factors, 54

**N**

NAC. *See* N-acetylcysteine
National Cancer Institute, 70
natural polyphenols, 41, 111, 117, 127
anticancer activities, 111–112
classes of, 111
as complementary medicine in
cancer therapy, 116
molecular targets of, 112–113
natural products, 18, 34–35, 69–72, 80,
81, 128, 129
as anticancer agents, 115–117
based drug discovery, 127
beta-elemene, 110
in cancer drug discovery, 128–129
curcumin, 114
economic impact of, 128–129
natural polyphenols. *See* natural
polyphenols
overcome multidrug resistance
with, 108–110
pterostilbene, 114–115
resveratrol, 113
tanshinones, 110
necrosis, 47
apoptosis and, 50
cross-talk among signaling
pathways in, 50
neurodegenerative diseases, 48

NF-jB, 52
NHDS. *See* non-herbal dietary
   supplements
Nijutsuto, 62
nobiletin, 23
   chemical structures, 134
non-herbal dietary supplements
   (NHDS), 90
nonsmall cell lung cancer (NSCLC), 115
non-steroidal anti-inflammatory drugs
   (NSAIDs), 102
novel agents, 18
novel compounds, 103–104
novel herbal extract, 32
novel natural products, 18, 35
NSAIDs. *See* non-steroidal anti-
   inflammatory drugs
NSCLC. *See* nonsmall cell lung cancer
nuclear factor erythroid 2-related
   factor 2(Nrf2), 44, 45
nuclear magnetic resonance (NMR), 37
nuclear transcription factor, 52

**O**

obesity, 87
onion. *See also Allium cepa*
   consumption, 93
   extracts, 93
   production, 93
*Oroxylum indicum,* 43
oxidative stress, 42, 45, 91
oxidized low-density lipoprotein
   (Ox-LDL), 89
Ox-LDL. *See* oxidized low-density
   lipoprotein

**P**

*Paeonia lactiflora,* 33
paeonol, 23
   chemical structures, 134

*Palmaria palmata,* 92
*Panax ginseng,* 34
PCA. *See* principal component
   analysis
PCa. *See* prostate cancer
*Pera benensis,* 18
*Persicaria capitata,* 100
persistent pain, 62
PG. *See* pharmacogenomics
P-gp. *See* P-glycoprotein
pharmaceutical development of
   potential cancer drugs, 123
pharmaceutical drug development, 81
pharmacogenomics (PG), 127
pharmacokinetics, 97
pharmacology, 67
phelligridins D, 26
   chemical structures, 134
phenolics
   benefits of, 89–90
   in healthcare products, 92–93
(poly)phenol metabolites, 88
phosphatase and tensin homologue
   (PTEN), 53
phosphorylation, 113
physcion-8-$O$-$\beta$-D-monoglucoside,
   37–39
   chemical structure of, 38
phytochemicals, 16, 31–32,
   34, 65, 68–69, 72, 75, 81,
   123, 126
   with antioxidative activity, 90–91
   based drug discovery, 129
   biotechnological production of, 126
   chemical structures of, 131–142
   from cruciferous vegetables, 5–8
   economic impact of, 128–129
   in herbal medicines, 1, 6
   metabolism of, 90
   molecular diversity, 127
   role in drug development, 70
   in vegetables and fruits, 6, 7
phyto-constituents, 42
phytotherapy, 68–69

picroliv, 22
PI3KCI-AKT-mTORC1, 53
piperine, 82
   chemical structures, 139, 141
piplartine, 82
   chemical structures, 139
plant-derived alkaloids, 70
plant-derived drugs, 70
plant extracts, anticancer activity of,
   18–19
plant molecules, 16, 43–44
   aglycones, 16–17
   anticancer activity
      ayurvedic medicinal plant with, 19
      of plant extracts and fractions,
      18–19
   costunolide, 19–21
   cynaropicrin, 19
   dehydrocostus lactone, 19, 20
   dioscin, 17–18
   ginsenosides, 17
   lappadilactone, 20
   with medicinal properties, 22–27
   C-17 polyene alcohol, 21
   *Saussurea costus. See Saussurea costus*
plant products, 42
plant secondary metabolites, 88
plasma concentration
   of genistein, 17
   of isoflavones, 17
platycodons, 17
podophyllotoxins, 76
C-17 polyene alcohol, 21
*Polygonum cuspidatum*, 31, 113
poly-L-lysine (PLL), 41
polyphenols, 89
pomiferin, 24
   chemical structures, 134
pomolic acid, 27
   chemical structures, 134
*Porphyra purpurea*, 90
*Porphyra* sp., 92
potent anticancer agents, 35

potential active anti-HSV
   molecules, 3
potential anticancer agents, 44, 107
potent natural products, 35
pregnane X receptor (PXR), 45
principal component analysis (PCA), 41
pro-apoptotic proteins, 51
pro-caspases-8–10, 50
programmed cell death, 47
   molecular mechanism of, 48–49
pro- or anti-apoptotic genes, 47
*Prosopis cineraria*, 91
prostate cancer (PCa), 67, 97
prostate-specific antigen (PSA), 90
proteinaceous anticancer agents, 43
protein kinase (PK)C inhibitor, 21
proteinomics, 70
protozoa, 2
PSA. *See* prostate-specific antigen
psychological stress, 30
PTEN. *See* phosphatase and tensin
   homologue
pterostilbene, 111, 114–115
pyrrolizidine alkaloids, 86

**Q**

Qi (pronounced "chee"), 8, 10
   deficiency in, 11
   distribution of, 11
quercitrin, chemical structures, 142

**R**

RA. *See* rheumatoid arthritis
RA-fibroblast-like synoviocytes
   (RA-FLSs), 36
RA-FLSs. *See* RA-fibroblast-like
   synoviocytes
randomized clinical trials (RCTs), 90
RCTs. *See* randomized clinical trials

receptor-interacting protein (RIP), 49
red grapes, 89
"red man syndrome", 97
Relinqing®, 100
respective active compounds, 3
resveratrol (Res), 31–32, 41, 111, 113
rheumatoid arthritis (RA), 36
*Rheum officinale*, 38, 39
Rhizoma Coptidis, 68
Rhizoma Corydalis, 31
Rhizoma Curcumae, 31
RIP. *See* receptor-interacting protein
RNA, 68
*R*-roemerine, 79
*Rohdea chinensis*, 80
rooperol, 24
    chemical structures, 135
rosemary extracts, 91
rosmarinic acid, 27
    chemical structures, 135

**S**

saikosaponins, 17
sakuranetin, chemical structures, 142
*Salvia miltiorrhiza*, 34, 110
*Sapindus rarak*, 91
sapogenol, 116
saponins
    in herbal medicine, 16
    medical application of, 2
*Sargassum* sp., 92
*Saussurea costus*, 3, 19
    active compounds from, 19–20
    cytostatic effects of, 20
    C-17 polyene alcohol, 21
    sesquiterpene lactones of, 20
*Saussurea lappa*, 19, 20
    costunolide, 21
    cynaropicrin, 21
    C-17 polyene alcohol, 21

SCLC. *See* small cell lung cancer
scopoletin, 26
    chemical structures, 135
*Scutellaria baicalensis*, 33, 34
seaweed biomass, 92
seizures, 96
SENL. *See* Supplement Energy and
    Nourish Lung
sesquiterpene lactones, 3, 19–21, 25
severe combined immunodeficiency
    (SCID) mice, 78
SGC7901/ADR cells, 68, 110
Shernovine, 76
signal transducer and activator of
    transcription 3(STAT3), 72, 114
skeletal muscle, 103
small cell lung cancer (SCLC), 67
small molecules, 71
small natural molecules, 104
soysaponins, 17
spiritual stress, 30
spirostanol saponin, 80
5β-spirost-25(27)-en-1β,3β-diol-1-
    *O*-α-lrhamnopyranosyl-(1→2)-
    β-D-xylopyranosyl- 3-*O*-α-
    lrhamnopyranoside (SPD), 80
STAT3. *See* signal transducer and
    activator of transcription 3
statins, 92
*Stephania pierrei* (Menispermaceae)
    cytotoxicity of, 79
    ethanol extract, 79
*Stephania tetrandra*, 109
steroidal saponins, 17
*Streptomyces peucetius*, 103
stress, 45
structure–function relationships, 1, 16
sulforaphane, 56
    chemical structures, 137
sulfur compounds, healthcare
    products with, 88–89
sulphoraphane, 24
    chemical structures, 135

Supplement Energy and Nourish Lung
(SENL), 109
syncope, 96
synthetic molecules, 35

# T

tamaractam, 36
  chemical structure of, 36
*Tamarix ramosissima*, 36
tamoxifen, 100
tanshinone IIA, 116
tanshinones, 110
targeted drugs, 69–71
  categories of, 71
  disadvantages, 71
targeted therapy, side effects, 71
taxanes, 31
Taxol, 43, 76
TCM. *See* Traditional Chinese
  Medicine
Teng-Long-Bu-Zhong-Tang (TLBZT), 33
ternatin, chemical structures, 142
theaflavin, 116
theophylline, 25
  chemical structures, 135
therapeutic products, with plant
  extracts, 90–91
TLBZT. *See* Teng-Long-Bu-Zhong-Tang
TNF-α. *See* tumor necrosis factor α
TNFR1. *See* tumor necrosis factor
  receptor-1
tocotrienol, 26
  chemical structures, 135
tonic treatment, 12
Traditional Chinese Medical Theory, 9
traditional Chinese medicine (TCM),
  6, 8, 17–19, 30–31, 61–62, 64–67,
  80, 86, 102, 123, 128
  and acupuncture, 11
  adjuvant cancer therapy with,
    124–125

anti-oxidant activity of, 9
in atherosclerosis treatment, 8
as complementary medicine for
  treatment, 9–10
complexity of research work, 126
in complex treatment regimens, 125
dietary supplements with, 90
and drug combination, 12
efficiency of, 9
essential part of, 9
evidence-based medicine, 62
and food plants, 9
formulations
  in cancer therapy, 63
  in medical strategy, 99
health benefits, 124
healthcare into diabetes care,
  62–63
healthcare products based on, 87
ingredients for food supplements, 32
phytochemicals from, 123
recent development on, 12–13
role in Western medicine, 65–66
supports and restores, 12
use of, 10
in Western medicine, 124
and Western therapeutics, 65
traditional herbal formulations, 33
transferase-mediated dUTP nick-end
  labeling (TUNEL), 36
transgenic models, 35
triglyceride, 89
*Trypanosoma brucei*, 78
tubeimosides, 17
tumor necrosis factor α (TNF-α), 20,
  37–39
tumor necrosis factor receptor-
  1(TNFR1), 37–39
tumor-related proteins, 70–72
tumors, development of, 11
TUNEL. *See* transferase-mediated
  dUTP nick-end labeling
type 2 diabetes, 98

# U

ULK1/2, 53
*Ulva* sp., 92
*Undaria pinnatifida,* 90
urinary tract infection (UTI), 100
UTI. *See* urinary tract infection

# V

vancomycin, 97
vascular endothelial growth factor
    (VEGF), 21
VEGF. *See* vascular endothelial growth
    factor
verbascoside, 26
    chemical structures, 136
vinblastine, 82
vinca alkaloids, 76, 115
vincristine, 82
*Viscum album,* 34

# W

Walker 256 tumor, 77
web-based Gene SeT Analysis Toolkit
    (WebGestalt), 67
WebGestalt. *See* web-based Gene SeT
    Analysis Toolkit

Western blot analysis, 31
Western medical treatment, 62
Western medicine, 30, 61, 64–67, 69
    co-administration of, 64–65
    traditional Chinese medicine in,
        65–66, 124
Western therapeutics, 65
wogonin, 23
    chemical structures, 136
World Health Organization, 18, 87

# X

xenograft models, 35

# Y

yanhusuo, 108
Yanhusuo San, 31
Yin-Yang
    deficiency in, 10, 11
    disorientation and imbalance of, 9
Yin-Yang balance, 66

# Z

*Ziziphus jujuba,* 33
Zyflamend, 32